CONTENTS

KETO DIET FOR BEGINNERS

INTERMITTENT FASTING

VEGAN MEAL PREP

KETO DIET

FOR BEGINNERS

Easy Everyday Low Carb Recipes

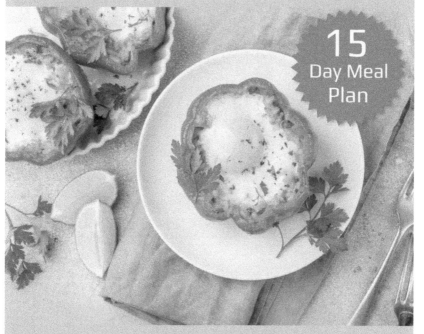

15 Day Meal Plan

Elyse Bose

INTRODUCTION

Big changes start off with simple things. By making a purchase of *Keto Diet for Beginners* you are making the first step on a chain reaction to a healthier lifestyle for you and your family. Whether you decide to take on Keto on your own or with a group or maybe just window-shopping for a new diet, this book will provide a good base. You don't even have to follow a Keto diet to benefit from the recipes in this book, which are all based on whole-foods, home cooking.

Chapter 1 will introduce you to Keto. It covers what the justifications for the diet are, and how low-carb diets work in general. It makes the case for swapping out sugar and high carbohydrate food for whole ingredients. The closer the ingredient is to its natural state, then the healthier it is. Adding sugars to products is the food industry's favorite way to get in your pockets and at the same time ruin your health.

Chapter 2 will go more in-depth about the hidden benefits of the diet, as well as cover some of the major caveats for those who wish to try Keto. Low-carb isn't for everyone and it is important you know what health considerations exist. Chapter 3 gives a full profile of the type of foods you will write down on your Keto shopping list. It also covers what alternatives exist, and what a typical Keto food pantry looks like.

Chapter 4 has some final tips and how-to's for maximizing Keto diet success. It can definitely be a hard diet, so these tips will guide you through any questions you have. Chapter 5 covers some excellent breakfast and lunch recipes for you to enjoy. Chapter 6 follows up with more substantial dinner recipes and chapter 7 provides some inspiration for snacks and Keto desserts. Finally, chapter 8 will list a full 15 days of eating on Keto, but you can modify it however you like.

HOW THE KETOGENIC DIET WORKS

IT IS no secret that the Ketogenic diet works wonders for weight loss. And it's become mainstream. Nowadays we hear people say, "I can't eat that because I'm on Keto", or they may wonder "Is x food Keto?" without even being on the diet. But they have heard so much about the diet from Instagram influencers to fitness professionals that they want to dabble in it. And why shouldn't they? Keto is the ideal diet plan for people who are a little too severely overweight. Keto can also work for the average Joe or fitness aficionado looking to stay slim yearlong.

So how does it work? All the magic happens on the plate (and to an extension, inside your body). Choosing a diet and meal plan that is high in low-carb, whole foods ingredients will decrease your waistline for as long as you stay on the diet. Some Keto believers even think that the days of counting calories are over! If you follow a low-carb diet meanwhile limiting your intake of processed foods, you are almost guaranteed to lose weight. Of course, if you put in the effort to count your calories, you stand to benefit from that as well. Keto is simply a diet you take on if you want to become healthier overall (not necessarily for weight loss)

Like any weight loss routine, all the power of Keto stems from the food itself. Regardless of your activity level or baseline weight, the diet works because you eat the right things. Consistency is really key here. Going on Keto only helps if you stick with it. One too many cheat meals may cause untold damage to your weight, or even reverse the progress from Keto. Unlike other diets, Keto makes it easy to follow a meal plan. There are many options, full of tasty ingredients that will have you looking forward to each meal.

The Power of Low-Carb

Keto is considered a low-carb diet. Typically, that means you will restrict carbohydrates anywhere from 100g to 50g daily. Sometimes this may go to 20g or even outright zero carbs. Carbohydrates are your enemy if you want to lose weight. This is difficult for some people to grasp, as carbs make up some of the tastiest foods you can imagine. Pizza, bagels, potato chips—these foods are all loaded with them. And they do tend to make us fat. Others will say that low-carb diets are unhealthy and that carbohydrates exist for a reason.

Of course, everyone is entitled to believe what they believe. The field of nutrition is one of the most hotly debated ones in health and wellness. Even among scientist and dietitians, they are strong opinions on many sides of the issue. It all comes down to the complexity of our biology—and the difficulty of testing weight loss diets experimentally. Some will say eat carbs (up to 60% of calories from carbohydrate sources) others will say that carbs should be limited (one of the first treatments for obesity in the 1800s was to cut back on carby foods).

We do know, however, that carbohydrates go hand in hand with fat storage. At the very least, carbohydrate foods are easy to binge on and lead to weight gain that way. Foods that are high in sugar (you know the ones) are also considered carbs. Perhaps one thing all dietitians can agree on is that sugar should be eaten in moderate amounts. There is a reason why most dieticians support a sugar tax on soft drinks. Products with high sugar content do cause weight gain, and in extreme cases may lead to the development of type 2 diabetes.

There is more contention when it comes to eating healthy carbs (whole-wheat grains, legumes, starchy vegetables). But the science tells us that all of these foods have one thing in common: they contain something called glucose, which is a type of sugar (or saccharide). As you may know, glucose that we get from our food travels into our bloodstream and provides our cells with energy. It gives your brain that extra kick you need to feel alert. This is why "carbing" up is a thing for many. By eating a high carb meal prior to exercise or an important exam at school you are giving yourself more energy.

But too much glucose is a bad thing, and that is what Keto tries to avoid. A moderate to high diet in carbohydrates is fine, but it is far too easy to overeat, especially when our pantries are full of Lays potato chips and Oreo brand cookies. When we eat too many carbohydrates we provide our body with more energy than it really needs. Not just in terms of calories, but in terms of glucose. Our bodies are efficient enough that they don't simply throw the extra away. Instead, it gets stored as adipose tissue or fat. This can either go under the skin (subcutaneous fat) which tends to collect in the hips, thighs and under the arms, or it can go to fat stores in the organs (visceral fat) which tend to collect around the base of the stomach.

And let's face—most of us are eating too many carbohydrates. It isn't really our fault either. The stuff is simply everywhere. Not all of us are able to make home cooked meals on a regular basis. Instead, we go for the easy stuff at fast food places or from snacks at the grocery store. This is less than ideal, as these meals are high in empty calories, most of them from carbs, sugar, and unhealthy fats. These foods are also higher in calories on average than healthier alternatives. Calories explode, and you end up gaining weight.

Most of these foods are also highly processed or highly refined, sometimes both. Any food that has more than three ingredients on the label is generally processed with additives, chemicals, and mechanical processes. Some of these processed foods have certain qualities that are bad for us. For example, white bread is a notoriously bad food because it is pure carbohydrate. Just like how sugar is "pure". When you eat them, they instantly get turned into glucose in the blood, and your blood sugar goes through the roof. This is also why fast food isn't filling. If you eat take out Chinese for dinner, you are hungry just a few hours later, which causes you to snack on other foods.

A low-carb, whole food based diet reduces blood sugar fluctuations. Not only is this healthier for you, but you will avoid the ups and downs of sugar crashes. What little glucose that does enter your body will go directly towards your energy needs—no stored food and no additional body weight to boot.

Making the switch to sugar-free, low-carb living is a no brainer. Everyone already knows that soda, candies, and other sugary foods are unhealthy. What most people don't realize is that the processed foods you buy at the store are also equally bad. These products are high in refined carbs plus they have high sugar content. Sugar or saccharides are often present (under several different names) in these products for taste and as a preservative.

But if you eat all your food from whole products, you never have to guess which ingredients are bad and which are good to eat. Mother Nature gives us all that we need. Under the Keto diet, you can enjoy all sorts of meat, veggies, and fruits. Bread is out of the picture, yet you can still enjoy copious amounts of dairy like milk and cheese. You can't drink any sugary drinks, but water is often all that you need. We all come from nature, so it makes sense to eat all natural foods.

Bad eating habits occur under our noses. First, it's one or two meals eating out and before you know it becomes a regular thing. This is the same as consistency but in the opposite sense. Instead of being consistently healthy you are consistently unhealthy.

hy Choose Keto?

The Ketogenic diet stands out because it is simple to follow. It has well-documented recipes and best practices for everyone. It doesn't matter if you are man or woman, overweight, obese, or completely healthy. Everyone benefits something from it. Some think that low-carb diets are just a fad. And while it is true that Keto popped out of nowhere during the 2010s, it isn't so much a fad as a lifestyle choice. People who start going on Keto also make healthier choices in general. If you are eating well and you feel good about it, you might also be doing yoga regularly or visiting the gym more often. For many, doing Keto isn't a fad but a dietary revolution.

The name Ketogenic comes from the metabolic process called Ketosis inside the body. It is what happens when you go low-carb (or zero-carb) for a long enough period. Since you don't get enough glucose from food to keep your engine running, the body decides to adopt an alternative fuel source. And that alternative fuel source is something we all have: Fat (sometimes in copious amounts). If glucose were gasoline, then the fat would be electricity running your car. It's much cleaner, much more efficient and it makes you feel good.

Not only that, but you will also lose weight. It's like hitting two birds with one stone—the ultimate weight loss diet. Imagine if somebody told you that you could take off chunks of fat from your body and use them to fuel your evening run?

Ketosis is a process in which fat gets converted into molecules called Ketone bodies (or Ketones for short). Like glucose, Ketones can be used by every cell in your body to do everything they need to do. This includes all the major organs and even your brain.

So no, cutting off carbohydrates isn't starving yourself or starving the brain. Not even close. We are robust enough that we can adapt to alternative energy sources when one runs out, even if it is by artificial means.

Usually one can just tell they are in Ketosis after a few days to a week of eating low-carb. You may first notice a general lull like you haven't eaten but after the Ketone bodies kick in you feel more energetic than ever before. Your mind clears up, and you feel unstoppable.

You can check for Ketone bodies manually by using different measures. The easiest is to use a product you breathe into that detects Ketone bodies in your respiration. Alternatively, you can use a blood meter and special "Keto sticks" to measure it.

In general, you don't have to do this though. After a week or so you will be in Ketosis. If you followed the meal plans at the end of this book then you can be sure of hitting Ketosis before the two weeks is over.

And here is where consistency shines. If at any point you decide you will cheat and have a little carby treat, you are taken out of Ketosis. The effect is almost instant. Generally, a cheat meal here and there will not disrupt long-term Ketosis, but you are definitely flirting with glucose. The body running on fat is different from the body running on glucose.

We are naturally primed to run on glucose, and for thousands of years, it has worked. But today we face a different challenge: a multi-billion food industry that wants to sell you easy to produce but god-awful food. We don't have to chase after our food anymore. Instead, it is on every street corner. We are getting fatter and dying from food-related diseases more than ever before.

Keto can help you prevent all that. Some would say that Keto comes at a steep price. Bread is just too good to give up... so is pasta, cake, and doughnuts. People who have been on Keto for years will say the opposite. They enjoy all the foods they eat on Keto and can't tell the difference in craving. They no longer get the mouthwatering reaction when they drive by a Dunkin Doughnuts or Cinnabon. Instead of sugar cravings, they get fat cravings, which will be explained a bit further on.

KETO DIET BENEFITS AND RISKS

CHOOSING any diet requires you to weigh the pros and the cons. No two diets are alike, and no two people will respond the same way to the diet. Some diets may be easier to follow for one individual but harder for another. For any diet to be an effective one it must have long-term sustainability. grain-based means that you are able to follow the diet requirements daily without turning to cheat meals or making a huge fuss about it.

While it is a healthy option, Keto does have its considerations. It has tons of benefits, too. Low-carb diets are not for everyone and neither are they the end of weight loss. But in a world of high sugar intake, rising diabetes and obesity rates, and even more commercial food products, Keto has its adherents.

Keto, as with all low-carb diets, aids with regulating your blood sugar levels. If you cut the intake of carbohydrates then you control the amount of extra blood sugar entering your body. This is good news for people who suffer from type 2 diabetes, obese, or who have pre-diabetes. Keto may effectively regulate your blood sugar levels to non-diabetic levels. It is worth talking with your doctor about making the switch, and whether they recommend it. Although it should be noted that Keto works like a therapy for diabetes, there is less evidence that it can reverse the disease. As soon as you eat that carby meal, your blood sugar is back to diabetic levels. Still, it's a good option.

Weight loss from Keto is to be naturally expected. You lose fat stores from Ketosis meanwhile keeping these stores low from lack of carbohydrates. Your body will slowly detoxify from high levels of sugar (if you are someone who comes from a high sugar diet). This is good news for our little friend the liver, who is responsible for metabolizing saccharides. Too much sugar consumption can cause liver problems, such as fatty liver disease.

Because visceral fat tends to collect around the abdomen, you can expect to lose fat in the same area. While there is no such thing as targeted fat burning through exercise, you can still achieve it through dieting. A body that is used to high sugar consumption may have tons of fat stored within organs themselves. Just like the fatty liver disease is a thing, so is fatty pancreas, gallbladder, and so on. Reducing carbohydrate intake will slowly melt the sugar in these organs, giving you a slimmer appearance about the waistline.

At the same time, you will benefit from the many dons of a whole foods diet. Vegetables come loaded with healthy fiber and vitamins and minerals. Keto dishes like bone broths and soups give you a full profile of the nutrients from meat and bones together.

Benefits of Ketosis

A body running on fat is a smarter body. Low-carb diets have been used for centuries to treat rare forms of drug-resistant epilepsy. For whatever reason, the loss of carbohydrates in the diet prevents seizures from occurring. This is a well-documented fact, and anyone who suffers from epilepsy should consider making the switch.

Our brains on fat, sometimes called the "fatty bran" (not to be confused with visceral fat like in fatty liver disease) also benefits. There is some evidence for example, that a Keto diet can help prevent neurodegenerative disease like Alzheimer's and Parkinson's. It also translates to better brain performance in general. Someone in Ketosis has a clearer, more focused mind. Their cognitive abilities are enhanced, which has been proven in animal and children studies.

Perhaps one of the more lucrative benefits of Ketosis is that you free yourself from the constant lows and highs of standard diets. You eat a high carbohydrate meal to fuel your next action, but in a few hours, your body will experience an inevitable crash. This crash, in turn, causes you to snack on food—a bad habit for weight loss. You ramp up the calories to match the decline in energy levels, but you end up gaining weight, especially if the snacks are unhealthy.

Keto promises a one-way ticket off the never-ending ride of the glucose cycle. Because glucose levels are stable throughout Ketosis, you don't feel the physical and psychological pressures to eat. Your energy levels will be at a constant high (except for when you have to sleep). Many athletes and fitness people chose the Keto diet and other low-carb diets for these reasons. There is never a precipitous drop in performance. And speaking about sleep, Ketosis also helps you sleep soundly. We aren't sure why, but it probably has something to do with the different brain biochemistry under Ketones.

The athletic benefits of Ketosis have been used both by bodybuilders and endurance athletes. Bodybuilders find that Keto allows them to build more muscle meanwhile lessening fat increase. Typically, muscle gain is followed by fat. The endurance athlete benefits because they are no longer limited by their natural glycogen stores in their muscles. Usually, once glycogen stores are used up we become exhausted and go no longer go on. This is called "hitting the wall" or the absolute limit of endurance training. If they are running on fat, they are less likely to experience this limitation.

Other Health Benefits

Keto diets may also help prevent the formation of cancer. Cancer cells are said to be "metabolically hyperactive" because of mutations in DNA. They don't know when to stop dividing and are constantly using up chemical energy to proliferate. Glucose is the obvious suspect. And if glucose is present in vast amounts, the cancer is free to leech off it after forming a blood supply.

The other major disease it may fight against is cardiovascular disease. This one is a major conundrum because Keto diets are typically high in fat. And fat has typically been related to an increased risk in heart disease. But, Ketosis regularly burns fat. Because blood glucose levels are stable, high blood sugar also goes down.

High blood sugar in diabetics causes arteries to constrict, further contributing to the risk of heart attack and stroke. On Keto blood sugar never gets very high so this risk is avoided. Keto can actually increase the level of good cholesterol HDL and lower bad cholesterol LDL. So if the high-fat content of Keto diets is worrying you, know that the fear is unfounded. Most of the fats you get from Keto will be heart healthy.

Because the diet is full of natural ingredients, it has anti-inflammatory properties. These can help treat or prevent arthritis, irritable bowel syndrome, and chronic pain. This is due to the effects of a major Ketone released during Ketosis called BHB. It is responsible for inhibiting the action of inflammation-causing compounds inside the body. For many, going Keto is the same as detoxifying from the various chemicals put in processed foods.

$\mathcal{R}$isks and Health Considerations

Upon first look, many will consider Keto a form of extreme diet. This is because of the carbohydrate content, which may be as low as 20g to 50g. The standard low-carb diet is billed at anywhere below 150g. With a little bit of experimenting, you can get 150g to 200g with a modified Keto diet. Usually by incorporating more legumes and starchy vegetables, but that is a far cry from the traditional version of Keto.

The low-carbohydrate content is worrying to some because of low blood sugar levels. If blood sugar drops completely you pass out and eventually die. It's something that diabetics are well aware of, as many diabetic treatments cause blood sugar to plummet. This risk is further increased by the possibility of developing Ketoacidosis—a condition characterized by elevated levels of blood Ketones. Ketoacidosis is more likely among diabetics and may present a medical emergency. It is critical that diabetics consult with their doctors first, and talk about which medications they are currently taking. Diabetics are recommended some level of medical supervision while going on the diet.

A lower carbohydrate consumption also naturally means a lower fiber intake. Couple this with a diet with an emphasis on fats and high animal proteins and you have the possibility of constipation. This can be alleviated with various forms of off the counter drugs, as well as prescription ones. But it's still largely preventable if you remember to get plenty of leafy greens and other veggies in your meals.

Low-carb diets have said to be difficult because of the way that they make you feel. And this is why some consider Keto to be an "extreme" diet. The symptoms you feel are the same ones you can expect from episodes of low blood sugar. They are symptoms that we all know well, even if we haven't been on low-carb diets before.

We feel hungry, tired, and irritable. Or at least, we feel that way for a little while. Normally these are cues that we have to eat something before we lash out at someone who is important to us. It is our brain's way of telling us that blood sugar levels are dropping. If we don't do anything to stop that decline, we may go into a low-blood-sugar episode resulting in loss of consciousness or even death.

Most people won't have to worry about any serious medical side effects from it, though. We have loads of extra glucose stored in our muscles and liver in the form of glycogen. When blood sugar levels go down glycogen is slowly melted to release glucose into the blood. While these symptoms probably won't do you much harm, they are still a bummer to get through.

Keto flu is a condition experienced during the first week or two of ditching carbs. Besides feeling the previously mentioned symptoms, you may also deal with flu-like symptoms. Think of it as a form of withdrawal from glucose. When addicts are trying to wean off drugs or alcohol they go through manic episodes. Their bodies rely so much on the drugs like our bodies rely so much on glucose that the absence of it shocks the body.

More distressing Keto flu symptoms may include nausea, vomiting, diarrhea, headache, dizziness, and muscle cramps. The presence of two or more of these symptoms will dictate if you are a good candidate for the diet. If these symptoms don't go away within a few days, or if the vomiting and diarrhea are constant, it is a sign that low-carb isn't for you, which is okay. Sometimes our bodies respond to the same stimulus in different ways. In these cases, it is better to err on the side of caution than to take unnecessary health risks,

For the vast majority of people, Keto is perfectly safe. Others who can't make it through the Keto flu may be suffering from an electrolyte imbalance or vitamin deficiency. There are ways to get around both. Even if you respond adversely to the diet at first, there are steps you can take to protect yourself against the risks. Some of these will be discussed in chapter 4.

But if you do make it through Keto flu without much difficulty, you are on your way to reaching Ketosis. A few days later and you might notice a slightly fruity odor coming from your mouth. This is evidence of the Ketone body acetone being present in your breath—a sure sign you are in Ketosis.

ULTIMATE KETO DIET SHOPPING LIST

KETO SUCCESS BEGINS with a carefully picked assortment of whole foods. The things you eat will directly influence how the diet works for you. When you go to the supermarket you will be bombarded by refined products with flashy announcements and enticing "healthy" labels. You need to ignore these unless they count as whole food. Everything else is marketing material. Focus your attention on the fresh produce aisle, the meat and frozen aisles, and lastly the dairy isles. Everything else is likely high in carbohydrates.

Whole foods are simple enough to spot. You can use the following formula at your discretion. Does it have an ingredient list? If no, it is probably a whole food product. If it does, are there 3 or fewer ingredients listed? If yes, then it is probably a whole food product. If there is more than 3, you will have to use your discretion. If it looks whole, then it probably is. However, if there is a slathering of different ingredients that you can't even pronounce, then don't touch that food with a five-foot pole.

After you determine something to be whole, ask yourself if the food falls in line with the philosophy of a low-carbohydrate Keto diet. If sugar is listed on the ingredient list, then you know that food is out. Next, if the food is high in carbohydrates then you can also rule it out. Remember low-carb is anywhere from 100g carbs a day to 50 and in extreme cases, as low as 20g or none at all. Considering that a medium sized apple alone has 25g carbs, you need to pick foods wisely. Otherwise, you will have a hard time staying in Ketosis, which is the whole point of the diet.

Keto requires a budget. Quality animal protein and fresh produce come at a cost. While cheaper alternatives are always an option, meat still tends to cost more than carby food. Most of the calories you consume will come from fat, though. Keto is traditionally low-carbohydrate, high fat with moderate protein consumption. The problem is that this protein needs to be sourced from fresh ingredients. Whereas before you could go to McDonald's or Chipotle and stock up on protein there, with Keto you have to cook most of your meals.

Meats

Animal proteins are the preferred protein source with Keto. They are high in vitamins, contain some fat, and are the highest protein foods. You can choose from red meats like beef, pork, and lamb and white meats like chicken and fish. Red meat tends to be higher in fat and protein but many are wary of it because of heart disease concerns. In that case, you could limit red meat or replace it entirely with white meat. It's still considered Keto and you can get plenty of protein from chicken and fish.

People on a strict Keto diet should avoid or severely limit their use of deli meats like ham, cured sausages, and bacon. Uncured sausage meat is fine. The cured varieties include things like pepperoni and salami. These products (as well as bacon) may come loaded with preservatives. If you can find such meats that are Keto friendly, then all the power to you. But usually, they are considered processed meat. The same goes for any beef jerky treat like slim Jims and so on. These are snack foods loaded with preservatives and should be avoided.

All chicken and fish are fair game. All seafood is game, including shrimps, scallops, ceviche, and shellfish. Canned fish such as tuna and sardines are also permissible. While technically processed meat, they are healthier than the cured meats mentioned above. They are also an excellent choice for doing Keto on a diet. But if you wish you don't have to buy canned meats. When it comes to Keto salmon is king. Not only does it taste good but it tends to be fattier than other varieties. Other fish choices include tilapia and trout.

Finally, don't underestimate the power of eggs. They are high in protein and healthy fats at once. You would be crazy not to eat them on your diet. They make natural breakfast and lunch foods, but can be enjoyed at all times of the day. They are also versatile. You can add an egg to virtually any meal to make it better.

Excellent Buys

- Ground beef (lean or fatty)
- Canned Tuna
- Salmon Fillet
- Sirloin steak cut
- Chuck Roast cut
- Chicken thighs and breast (with or without bones, with or without skin)
- Whole chicken or rotisserie chicken
- Trout and tilapia fillets

- Frozen shrimp
- Flank steak
- Round steak
- Pork shoulder
- Pork loin roast
- Pork spare ribs
- Pork sirloin
- Eggs

*V*egetables

Another staple of Keto is green veggies. These are either starchy (white potatoes, squash, etc.) or non-starchy (spinach, kale, cauliflower, broccoli, cabbage, carrots, green beans, etc.). Non-starchy vegetables are your primary targets. Avoid all starchy vegetables as they are high in carbs. If you really like potatoes, you can switch them out for rutabaga or sweet potatoes which have lowered carbs. Each vegetable will have a fiber content in addition to total carbohydrate. For calculating your Keto macros, you will use "net-carbs" or total carbohydrate minus the total fiber. Use this number to calculate how much you can eat towards your carb limit.

*V*egetables aren't very high in calories. You can eat one or two cups of leafy greens in one sitting and only consume some 50 or 60 calories. This is by design, as veggies were meant to be slathered with butter, olive oil, and other high-fat condiments. This is where most of your calories will come from.

Excellent Buys

- Spinach, kale, collard greens
- Cabbage, lettuce, bok choy, romaine lettuce
- Zucchini, cucumber, eggplant, okra
- Avocado (though technically a fruit)
- asparagus, chard, jicama, celery
- Anything that is green, or has green leaves and is low carb

Fruits

Tread with caution when picking out fruit. The naturally sweet flavor comes from a sugar called fructose. Many fruits are high in it, and as a consequence, they are high in carbohydrates. Apples are notoriously sweet but come at a high carbohydrate cost per serving. Other fruits like watermelon and cantaloupes are extremely carby. A whole medium-sized watermelon may contain up to 400 total carbohydrates. As such, you should look up the carbohydrate content of each fruit before you decide to eat it. Low-carb Keto discourages many fruits but doesn't ban them outright. After all, they are considered whole foods. Because they are high in carbs, some people on Keto simply won't eat apples, bananas, and various other carby fruits.

Berries are considered a fruit but are low in carbs. So are oranges and a few others. It's not that you can't eat fruit outright—you just need to eat the right fruits

Excellent Buys

- Avocados
- Olives
- Coconut
- Blackberries

- Raspberries
- Strawberries
- Tomatoes
- Lemons (and other citruses)

Dairy and Fats

The bulk of your caloric intake will come from either fat or dairy. For those that can't eat dairy, there are still many options to choose from. Cooking with a fatty oil like butter, olive oil, and coconut oil is the way the go. So is buying fatty cuts of meat or deciding to keep the skin on your meat (and eating it). In a pinch, nuts can also deliver fatty goodness but they tend to be high in carbohydrate so be careful with portion sizes.

Look for cooking oil that is unrefined. This means you can't use vegetable oils like canola oil. If you want to be safe, stick to extra-virgin olive oil, coconut oil, avocado oil and various types of nut oils. Be wary that these unrefined oils have a lower smoking point than the vegetable oils you may be used to. This means you will be burning oil long before you cook your food if the recipe requires a high temperature like stir-fried dishes. This is one of the reasons why many Keto recipes require you to use an oven. You just aren't going to get high-temperature output using olive and coconut oil. Butter and animal lard are also highly encouraged.

. . .

*D*on't be afraid of fat. Embrace all fat that is healthy to drive up your Ketosis progress. Do not buy products that are labeled with "low-fat" they usually have high sugar or alternative sweetener content.

*E*xcellent buys

- Avocados (again)
- Any whole, or shredded cheese (Parmesan, cheddar, jack)
- Coconut oil
- Extra virgin olive oil (unrefined
- Cottage Cheese
- Diary Creams (sour, heavy, whipped)
- Nuts and seeds (raw)
- Butter

*F*oods to Avoid

Anything not listed above is strictly not allowed. But if you want to have a modified or lenient version of Keto nothing is stopping you. You will, however, struggle to get into Ketosis as quickly (or at all) if you eat too many carbohydrates. In tradition with the whole-foods movement, most processed foods are out of the question. But if you decide to eat some every now or then or even regularly, nothing is stopping you. As long as you limit these things, and still lead with a majority whole-foods based approach, then this is okay. Only the most pedantic Keto people will tell you not to eat canned tuna or canned anything. Or that you should make homemade alternatives to every little ingredient like mayonnaise, mustard, seasonings and so on. Sometimes it is worth purchasing a processed food if it pays off in terms of convenience and overall adherence to the diet.

*C*arby foods that may still be considered healthy are also off limits because they can bring you out of Ketosis. This means no bread or legumes or products derived from them. No pasta, for example. And since peanut butter is made from peanuts (which are a legume) it is also prohibited. People are often surprised to hear this because peanut butter is a fatty spread high in protein and overall really good for you. Sadly, it isn't Keto. As an alternative, you can try using various nut butters which is the same thing more or less, but made out of nuts (rather than a legume). These do pack a high carbohydrate profile though, and should be limited.

*S*alt and pepper are considered Keto. Any other seasoning bought from the store should be taken in with a grain of salt (pun intended). Usually, if the seasoning or spice is sourced from natural ingredients and doesn't have a bunch of additives then it is perfectly okay to use it.

*F*inally, absolutely no sugar. By extension, no sugar alternatives either. Anyone who tells you that coke zero is Keto is teetering on the edge between eating for pleasure and still trying to lead a healthy lifestyle. This is a major area of contention where you must make the final decision. Many Keto sweets and desserts are made using artificial sweeteners and many enjoy them. But all of these sweeteners are still processed foods and they clash with the Keto ideal. While artificial sweeteners do not have any carbs, they have been linked with loads of nasty things like increased risk of cardiovascular disease, weight gain, and high levels of insulin.

A word about protein shakes. While massively popular even with the Keto crowd, these products are still technically a type of processed good. Whether or not you decide to use them is up to you. Virtually any protein shake powder that has a flavored component is using either sugar or an alternative sweetener. If you look at most flavored protein shake labels you will see a long list of ingredients. Compare this with an unflavored version, which may only have 3 or four ingredients. You can get all the protein that you will ever need from eating quality meat products at each meal.

*I*f you absolutely must have your protein, be wary of the brand you chose. Always pick the unflavored kind (throw in some berries or butter for taste). Do your research. Some powders are healthier than others. This may come at a cost, but you pay a premium for things that are good for you. Since protein powders are consumed regularly, this is not a product you want to go cheap on.

The No Buy List

- Sugar or products containing it (check the label)
- Grain or grain-based food (cereal, bread, pasta, baked goods, etc.)
- Processed foods and snacks (if it comes in a box, throw it out)
- Sugary drinks and candy (including all energy drinks, healthy fruit juices, and sweetened teas)

- Most type of fast food (check the nutritional information for carbs and sugar)
- Ice cream or other frozen treats that are not Keto
- Chocolate (unless dark chocolate)
- Pizza
- Meal replacements, protein shakes and so on

TIPS FOR KETOGENIC SUCCESS

LET'S FACE IT, Keto isn't easy. The rules may be easy, and recipes may taste good and be easy to make, but you will still feel that something is missing. And this feeling will persist long after you are in Keto. Usually, it goes away after a long time of being on Keto and reaching what some call fat "acclimation". But that's not much of a science.

In the meantime, you will have to resist carbohydrate and sugar cravings all the time. If you have difficulty following the diet you will inevitably fail. No, you won't be starving. But your body will try to convince you that you are in the beginning. The low-blood sugar response will always be nagging at you until blood sugar levels eventually stabilize.

But before that happens, here are some tips to ensure your maximum success, both in terms of staying on the diet and being healthy while you do it.

. . .

*E*at Salt

No, salt won't kill you. And if you are doing Keto you will need lots of it. Being on Keto puts you in a natural state of sodium loss. The kidneys will excrete sodium at a quicker rate than before. Loss of sodium may result in undesirable symptoms like nausea, lightheadedness, fatiguing, and especially muscle cramps. So whenever you get the chance, make sure that you pour on the salt. And you can do so without feeling any guilt.

*S*tay Hydrated

Water is your friend. Coffee and tea are your friends. Ignore all the rest. These are the three things you are allowed to drink, as anything else will have either sugar, high carbohydrate content or artificial sweeteners. While dairy is allowed, milk is too carby to also be allowed. You might be surprised how far you can get with just water, coffee, and tea.

Though coffee is a diuretic it doesn't really dehydrate you—you just pee more often. Big deal. If plain water is boring you can dry mineral water, water fruit infusions (leave the pulp) or lemon and cucumber water.

If you are on a low-carb diet you will naturally lose more water than usual because glycogen stores retain water. As you go into Ketosis, these stores get used up, and less water is kept in your body.

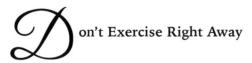

*D*on't Exercise Right Away

The transition to Keto will be slow at first. Treat it as recovering from surgery: no strenuous exercise for 2 weeks at least, or until you have recovered. Getting into Ketosis may take up to a week or even more. If you do decide to exercise, stick to low-intensity walking and never for distances greater than 3 miles. At this stage, your body is very sensitive to glycogen depletion. Your glucose stores are low and have yet to stabilize. Exercising would be asking for trouble. You are likely to experience heat stroke, loss of consciousness or even death from an episode of low blood sugar. If you are a diabetic the warning is doubly so.

Remember that athletes regularly "carb-up" before doing their workouts. Before you are in Ketosis there is no way you can do this. Carbing up will delay Ketosis, further contributing to failure on the diet. The best thing to do is wait a little bit until your body is used to Keto.

The Ketogenic diet does not prohibit working out—quite the contrary. If you are burning fat for energy you can expect increased performance in the gym or out on a hike.

Note Your Electrolyte Balance

Electrolytes are those things that you get from drinking Gatorade. More specifically, they are compounds in your body that play a vital role in maintaining balanced systems throughout like regulating temperature and hormonal activity. A loss of electrolytes can make you feel bad, or even cause death. You naturally lose them through sweating so they go hand in hand with dehydration. Both sodium and potassium are types of electrolytes and are most at risk of plummeting during Keto. You lose them because your kidneys regularly flush them out on a low-carb diet, because you lose water weight on the diet, and because you can't eat many potassium-rich foods like beans.

Besides eating lots of salt, some veggies can give you all the potassium that you need, so make sure you are eating them regularly.

*D*on't Underestimate the Role of Sleep

Because fatigue and irritability are common symptoms of the Keto flu, you can't rule out the possibility that these things are due to lack of sleep. If you are an adult you need a full 7 to 8 hours of good, quality sleep each night. Sleep deprivation may further contribute to negative symptoms by releasing the stress hormone cortisol.

Instead of playing an endless guessing game to determine where your symptoms are coming from, it is better to eliminate causes one by one.

A lack of sleep means there is something wrong with your schedule (either too much work or too much entertainment seeking) or that you are having physical and psychological problems falling asleep.

Avoid drinking caffeine after dinner. Get regular exercise to exhaust yourself before bed and unplug from technology 30 minutes before bedtime.

*E*at at Your Caloric Requirement

Obviously, eating fewer carbohydrates will reduce your overall calorie consumption. This means that during the first days of the diet you may be tempted to eat less than you normally would. This is calorie restriction which by itself will make you feel tired and irritable most of the time. If you aren't trying to lose weight then try to eat a little more calories. You can do this by increasing portion sizes or adding more meals.

KETO BREAKFAST AND LUNCH RECIPES

START the day off right with a healthy Keto breakfast or lunch. These recipes are what you would expect from traditional breakfast meals but without all of the carbs. Instead of reaching for the refined carbs pick up the healthy fats and proteins. Throw in a few veggies and you have yourself a made breakfast. As with all Keto recipes, feel free to get creative with your meals. Who wants to eat plain old scrambled eggs every morning (not that there is anything wrong with that). Consider boiled eggs, frittatas, or wiping up some delicious deviled eggs.

Easy Breakfast Platter

Sometimes the best breakfast is the simplest one. By putting together lots of different whole foods in a single dish you diversify your meal and hit whatever macro requirements you are looking for.

. . .

Ingredients

- 4 – 6 bacon strips
- ½ cup Brussels sprouts
- 3 eggs boiled
- Half an avocado
- Plum tomato (sliced or whole)

Preparation

Requires minimal cooking. Cook bacon on a pan and gently roast the Brussels sprouts until browned. Cut avocado into thin slices. Add salt and pepper for seasoning. Cut boiled eggs into half's if preferred put all ingredients in a large plate and enjoy.

Ghee

A traditional butter from India. Works as an excellent butter or oil substitute in all your Keto dishes.

Ingredients

- 1lb. regular butter

Preparation

Let the butter melt in a pan using low heat.

Allow the heat to simmer to a low, and leave butter alone for about an hour. Look out for a foam to form along with the pan.

Underneath the foam should be a type of milky white substance. This is milk protein from the butter. It isn't needed for the ghee, which is pure butterfat.

Get a jar or whatever container you wish to store your Ghee in. Carefully filter out the milk protein using a coffee filter or cheese-cloth. The milk protein should stay behind, and the butterfat should be the result.

Makes about 1 cup of Ghee.

Bullet Proof Coffee

*Y*ou may have heard of this one already. All it is, is coffee made the Keto way. An excellent way to jump-start your day.

*I*ngredients

- 2 tbsp. regular butter or Ghee
- 1 tbsp. MCT oil or coconut oil (avocado and nut oils can be used too)
- And a cup of coffee of course!

*P*reparation

The easiest way to make the final blend is by using a blender. Add all the ingredients together and give it a few whirls.

Alternatively, you can try stirring the ingredients in with a spoon, but this is often ineffective.

Guacamole Breakfast Stack

*E*ggs, guac, and sausage. What else could you ask for in a breakfast?

*I*ngredients

- 1 avocado (pitted)
- ½ small onion chopped
- 2 tbsp. fresh lime juice
- 6 oz. gluten-free ground sausage meat
- 2 eggs
- Salt and pepper for taste
- 2 tsp. Ghee

*P*reparation

Make the guac by adding avocado, chopped onion and lime juice in a small bowl. Mix and mash until desired consistency is reached.

Add ghee to a pan for frying the sausage. Cook sausage in small paddies. Two minutes per each side. When done, fry two eggs, sunny side up. Add more ghee if needed.

Finally, using the sausage patty as a base, add a layer of guacamole and top it off with the eggs. The end result should look like a burger. For better results, use a circular egg ring to prevent the eggs from spilling to the sides of the pan

Cauliflower Breakfast Toast

*A*n egg-based breakfast toast. Ideal for eating alone or with additional toppings.

*I*ngredients

- 1 head cauliflower
- 1 large egg
- ½ shredded cheddar cheese (or your choice of cheese)
- 1 tsp. garlic powder
- Salt and Pepper

*P*reparation

Preheat oven to 425 degrees and get a baking sheet ready with parchment paper. Use a cheese grater to finely grate the cauliflower and place contents in a microwave-safe bowl. Microwave the bowl for around 8 minutes, drain with paper towels if necessary.

Crack an egg into cauliflower bowl, add cheese, and garlic powder a swell. Season with salt and pepper. Mixed until evenly distributed. Then make toast sized patties out of the mixture. Spray baking sheet with cooking oil and place patties on top. Bake until toasty, around 18 to 20 minutes.

Add any Keto friendly toppings you wish, including heavy cream, more eggs, bacon, guacamole, or veggies.

Mushroom Omelet

a quick to whip up meal, ideal for breakfast or lunch. But who cares, you can eat it anytime.

I ngredients

- 3 eggs
- 1 oz. butter or Ghee
- 1 oz. shredded cheese (of your choosing)
- 1 oz. yellow onion
- 3 mushrooms sliced
- salt and pepper

P reparation

Whisk eggs in mixing bowl until evenly distributed. Add salt and pepper at this time. Add butter to frying pan on medium to high heat and wait for butter to fully melt. Then pour eggs on the pan. Wait for the omelet to form on the bottom but not yet fully cooked on top. Add the cheese, mushrooms, and onions.

The final part is the trickiest. When the bottom seems sufficiently cooked, use a spatula to fold it over the top. Be careful not to accidentally cause a tear in the omelet. Then when it has gotten golden brown underneath you can remove it from the pan and enjoy

Serves 1

Breakfast Tuna Platter

. . .

*I*deal for those mornings or afternoons when you want to get more protein in. You can be sure that these ingredients are all fresh and whole foods.

*I*ngredients

- 4 eggs
- 2 oz. spinach or other leafy green
- 10 oz. tuna in olive oil (canned okay, make sure it is Ketogenic)
- 1 avocado
- ½ cup Keto Caesar dressing
- salt and pepper

*P*reparation

Boil eggs for 4 to 8 minutes. A softer boil will require less time in the water. For easier shell removal, cool eggs in cold water immediately after removing them from the boiling water. Cut eggs into halves and season to your preference.

Add spinach to a bowl, slice the avocado into thin pieces, and place the eggs with them. Add the tuna to make one happy looking platter. Serve with a side of Caesar dip or plain mayonnaise.

Serves 2

Sirloin Steak Salad

. . .

A quick and easy salad for mid-afternoon lunch. Remember to use the freshest ingredients. The use of olive oil is optional but will add some healthy fats to the steak.

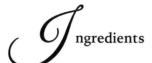

Ingredients

- 1 Pound sirloin steak
- 2 tbsp. Olive oil
- 2 Romaine Lettuce Hearts
- 3 eggs, hard-boiled diced
- 2 Avocados diced in large chunks
- 2 cups cherry tomatoes
- 3 tbsp. Keto Caesar Dressing

Preparation

Season steak with your choice of spices. Salt and pepper work well. Warm up a pan with 2 tbsp. of olive oil. Sear both sides of steak for around 2 minutes each. Let steak sit for 10 minutes. Note that olive oil burns at low temperature. The steak will have a somewhat medium consistency.

After it has sat for 10 minutes, cut the steak into thin slices. Add steak, veggies, and eggs into large salad bowl and mix. Add Caesar dressing and enjoy.

Serves 2 – 4

Keto Caesar Dressing

. . .

A fatty Caesar dressing you can use on all of your salads or as a dip or side for various meals. Note that this recipe is high in healthy fats.

Ingredients

- 3 garlic cloves minced (finely)
- 1 ½ tsp. anchovy paste
- 1 tsp. Worcestershire sauce
- 2 tbsp. lemon juice (around half a lemon)
- 1 ½ tsp. Dijon mustard
- ¾ cup mayo
- Salt and pepper for taste

Preparation

Mince the garlic (use a garlic press to save time). You can use a heavy knife as well. To garlic add the anchovy paste, Worcestershire sauce and lemon juice to a small bowl. Whisk well. Add mayo to the mix and whisk until everything is evenly distributed. Ready to serve. Store in the fridge, in a large cup or jar.

Cauliflower Mac & Cheese

A low-carb alternative to the traditional mac n cheese dish.

. . .

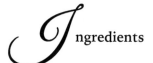

Ingredients

- 1 full head of cauliflower
- 1 cup cheddar cheese
- 3/4 cup heavy cream
- Salt and Pepper

Preparation

Break apart cauliflower with hands or cut with a knife into small chunks. Boil in water for 5 minutes on high. Drain and add salt and pepper to cauliflower. Add heavy cream and mix together. Add cheddar cheese and mix. Serve with your choice of herbs and garnishes.

Serves 2 – 4

Lemon Butter Chicken

A great afternoon meal packed with protein and taste

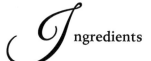

Ingredients

- 1 lb. boneless chicken breast (skinless for leaner meat, with the skin on for more fat content)
- Lemon pepper
- 1 tbsp. extra virgin olive oil (or just virgin)
- ½ stick of butter

- 3 garlic cloves minced
- 2 lemons (for juice) and the zest of one
- ¼ cup heavy cream
- ½ cup small cherry tomatoes

*P*reparation

Season chicken with lemon pepper and salt. Heat oil in medium-high heat (skillet or pan). Sear chicken until browned and well cooked throughout. Around 10 minutes per side. Remove chicken from the pan and make the sauce on the same pan. You should have some residue from the cooked chicken and lemon pepper. Leave it as is.

Place butter in a pan and let it melt. Add garlic, stir for around one minute, and then add lemon juice and zest. Add the cream next and bring the pan to a simmer. Add cherry tomatoes and lemon slices. Let simmer for another 5 minutes and then put the chicken back into skillet.

Serve with your choice of leafy greens.

Serves 2 – 4

Cheese and Steak Filled Peppers

*T*his recipe goes down well as either a breakfast or lunch. Either way, it will satisfy all of your cheesy and meat cravings with a good amount of fiber too.

. . .

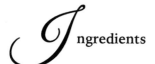

Ingredients

- 4 medium bell peppers, with seeds removed, cut into halves
- 1 cup cut onion (thinly sliced)
- 1 cup mushrooms (thinly sliced)
- 1 tbsp. olive oil
- 1 lb. sirloin steak, cut into thin slices before getting cooked
- Salt and pepper.
- Provolone slices (two per pepper half)

Preparation

Preheat oven to 325 degrees. Bake peppers for 30 minutes. Prepare a pan or skillet with olive oil and bring the heat to a medium-high. Add onions and mushrooms and let simmer for 1 minute. Add salt and pepper at this time. Add the sirloin steak and add even more salt and pepper (not too much, but enough to season the steak). Cook everything for about 3 minutes.

One by one, add a provolone slice to each pepper once out of the oven. Add a generous amount of steak and mushroom onions you made previously to each pepper. Be careful not to add too much. Place it gently on top of the first provolone slice. Add yet another provolone slice on top of the meat.

Finally, broil in the oven for another 3 minutes or until cheese is melted to your liking. Serve with your choice of additional toppings or Keto friendly sauce.

Serves 2 – 4

KETO DINNER RECIPES

IN THE STANDARD three-meal diet dinner is usually the biggest meal you have all day. It is no different if you are on a Keto diet. Ideally, each dinner plate should consist of one high protein cut of meat, poultry, or fish alongside a generous helping of non-starchy vegetables. The meat or fish should be prepared in such a way that gives you lots of fat. A common problem with beginner Keto people is that they wonder from where all their fat comes from. You already learned about this in chapter 3 but it bears repeating here. Add fatty sauces, creams, and oils to your meals whenever possible. Add dairy. If you don't have a favorite cheese as of yet now is the time to pick one, because you will be seeing a lot of it in your meals.

*B*ut since there are many different types of animal proteins and many types of vegetables to choose from, you can still think of clever dishes to whip up. Here just a few for inspiration.

Pork Chops with Green Beans and Avocado

A well-balanced dinner with a little bit everything. A little bit of fat, veggies, and protein for your liking.

Ingredients

- 1 tbsp. chipotle paste
- 2 tbsp. olive oil
- Salt and pepper
- 8 oz. pork chops (can use multiple)
- 10 oz. green beans
- 2 avocados
- 5 scallions
- 4 oz. butter
- 1 garlic clove

Preparation

Make a marinade using the chipotle paste, olive oil, and salt in a small bowl. Fully cover the meat in jump-start marinade and leave aside for 15 minutes. Or for a longer marinade do so in a plastic bag left for 30 minutes in the fridge.

Preheat oven to 400 degrees and grill the meat on a baking sheet. Leave in oven for 20 – 30 minutes, turning at 10 to 15 minutes. While you wait get garlic butter and green beans ready. Mine or press the garlic and mix in with butter and pepper. Add additional spices like paprika if you'd like. Set aside to eat with the rest of the dish.

Get a frying pan going with some olive oil. Raise heat to medium-high. Place green beans in a pan and sauté for 5 minutes. As green beans come to an end, lower heat slightly to add spices.

Finely cut scallions and prepare avocados. Mix both of them in with the scallions but mash the avocado first with a spoon. Remove pork from oven and you are ready to enjoy. Oven grilling is completely optional—but it is convenient. Nothing is stopping you from frying it on a pan.

Sausage Alfredo with Zucchini Noodles

*W*ho said you can't have pasta on Keto? Well everyone—pasta isn't allowed. But you can still try these zucchini noodles with Alfredo sauce to kick away your pasta cravings.

*I*ngredients

- 8 – 12 ounces gluten-free sausage ground
- 2 tbsp. butter or Ghee
- 3 cloves garlic
- 1 cup heavy cream
- ½ cup grated Parmesan
- Salt and pepper
- 2 zucchini specialized

*P*reparation

Cook with sausage in a large skillet using medium

heat. Let cook until sausage is brown. Takes around 5 to 8 minutes. Put the sausage on a plate and leave the skillet for the next step. Add butter and let melt to the same pan, followed by adding the garlic. Make sure garlic is minced either by hand or using a mincer. Let simmer for about one minute stirring occasionally.

Next, add the heavy cream and reduce the heat until it is nice and thick. Stir when needed.

Add the parmesan after 5 to 8 minutes. Use salt and pepper for taste. Then add the sausage, making sure to mix everything well.

For the zucchini noodles, you can either buy some that spiralized already from the store or you can do it yourself. Having a spiralizer handy is the easiest way to do it, but you can also do it with other tools. Place these in a microwave safe bowl and heat for around 2 minutes. They will be tender to the touch when done. Add the sauce you made to the noodles and enjoy.

Serves 2 – 4

Fried Salmon, Broccoli, and Lemon Mayo

*T*his recipe packs a zesty taste along with a healthy dose of fats and proteins

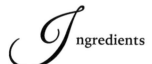

*I*ngredients

- 1 cup mayo
- 8 - 16 oz. salmon
- Salt and pepper
- 1 lb. broccoli

ELYSE BOSE

- 2 oz. butter
- 2 tsp. lemon juice

*P*reparation

Get a bowl and mix the mayonnaise and lemon juice together. For a fattier meal, you can also add some heavy cream into the mix.

Cut the salmon into smaller, pieces. For most people, 8 oz. is a little high. Cut into 4 oz. if you prefer or keep serving size at 8 oz. for a meal that is extra high in protein.

Get a pan going with the butter just barely melted on medium heat. Fry salmon for a few minutes each side, making sure to bring down the heat as it cooks.

Rinse broccoli and cut out stems. Alternatively, use tiny or frozen broccoli. Keep pieces small.

There should be butter left over in pan from the salmon (if not, add another ounce or so). Add broccoli and bring the heat to medium-high for a few minutes until broccoli is browned. Season to your liking and stir butter good.

Serve the salmon, lemon mayo and broccoli together.

Serves 2 – 4

Cabbage Noodle Beef Stroganoff

*I*nstead of noodles, this stroganoff uses the low-carb version (cabbage). It doesn't sacrifice any taste, though.

· · ·

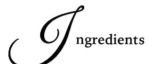

Ingredients

- 1 ½ lb. sirloin sliced into thin pieces
- 1 tbsp. tomato paste
- 5 tsp. butter
- 1 large head of cabbage (about 1 lb.) thinly sliced
- salt and pepper
- 2/3 cup sour cream
- 8 oz. mushrooms thinly sliced
- ½ red onion sliced thin
- ¾ beef broth

Preparation

Get about 3 tsp. of butter and add it to a large skillet or pan. Bring heat to medium-high until butter is fully melted. Then add the mushrooms with salt and pepper. Sauté the mushrooms for about 5 minutes (they should be brown) then move them to a separate bowl.

Lightly season beef with salt and pepper. Add it to the pan (still hot) and cook until well done. Allow some 5 to 8 minutes for it to cook and add it with the mushrooms.

Now sauté the onion in the same bowl. If there isn't enough butter then add 1 tbsp. more. Mix in tomato paste and add the broth (homemade or store bought). Then let simmer. Leave about a ½ cup of broth at least.

In a separate bowl, mix sour cream with a ½ cup of the broth. Stir it well, and then add sour cream back into the pan. Return the beef and mushrooms to the pan and stir well.

In a large pot, melt 2 tsp. of butter and then add cabbage, salt pepper and about 2 tbsp. of water. Make sure heat is on medium high.

Leave on low heat until cabbage fully cooked then put on top of the stroganoff

Serves 2 – 4

Low-Carb Traditional Beef Stew

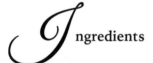his dish takes a couple of hours to complete but is well worth it in the end. Depending on the tenderness of the meat, your mileage may vary.

ngredients

- 1 ¼ pound beef chuck roast in cubes (about 1 inch)
- 2 - 3 celery stalks sliced
- 8 oz. whole mushrooms, cut into quarters
- 4 oz. onions diced
- 3 oz. carrots sliced or roll cut
- 2 garlic clove sliced
- 2 tbsp. olive oil
- 2 tbsp. tomato paste
- 5 cups beef broth (homemade or store bought)
- 1 large bay leaf
- salt and pepper

$\mathcal{P}$reparation

Chuck roast can be either fatty cuts or lean. If so desired, trim extra fat off. Wash vegetables and clean everything before chopping. Put everything in a bowl including garlic. Mix olive oil into the beef,

Sear beef in a large pot in small batches if necessary. Add oil as tilapia. Once all of it browned, add all of the beef into pot and stir in bay leaf and tomato paste. Beef should be well marinated. Let cook for less than a minute and add a cup of broth. Make sure you scrape beef off the floor of the pot if it has stuck. Adding the rest of the broth bring the stew to a low simmer and cover. Let cook for 1 ½ hour, or until beef has desired tenderness.

Tender meat should be easy to put a fork through with little resistance. Once tender, add vegetables, and raise the heat slightly. Once simmering, bring the heat down and let cook uncovered for another 40 minutes until vegetables fully cooked. Add salt and pepper.

Makes 4 to 7 servings

Chicken Noodle Soup (without the noodles)

$\mathcal{T}$hink like the chicken noodle soup your mom used to make, but with a low-carb twist!

$\mathcal{I}$ngredients

- 6 oz. mushrooms sliced
- A full chicken, shredded, (rotisserie chicken for ease)

- 2 celery stalks
- 2 garlic cloves minced
- 2 cup green cabbage shredded into thin strips
- 4 oz. butter
- 2 tbsp. dried onion (minced)
- 1 carrot
- 8 cups chicken broth (homemade or bought from the store)
- Salt and pepper

$\mathcal{P}$reparation

Slice celery and mushrooms into tiny pieces. Add butter to a large pot. Turn on heat to medium-high until butter is fully melted. Mince garlic using a press.

Add onion, mushrooms, celery, and garlic to the pot and let cook for a few minutes. Then add the broth along with sliced carrots and parsley. Let cook until vegetables are tender.

Finally, add the shredded chicken (should already be cooked) and cabbage. Let simmer for another 8 to 12 minutes until cabbage looks tender.

Serves 2 – 4

Pesto Salmon with Spinach

$\mathcal{E}$asy to make dinner with a side of leafy greens. Pesto flavor leaves the dish tasting savory.

· · ·

Ingredients

- 25 oz. salmon
- 1 lb. spinach or baby spinach
- 2 tbsp. butter, Ghee or olive oil
- salt and pepper
- 1 tbsp. green pesto
- 1 cup mayonnaise, sour cream or heavy cream
- 2 oz. shredded cheese (your choice)

Preparation

Preheat oven to 400 degrees. Get a baking dish ready, using butter or oil. Lightly season salmon fillet with salt and pepper and place on a baking dish. If fillets have skin, place with the skin facing down.

Add mayonnaise, pesto, and your choice of cheese to the fillets. Bake for around 20 minutes. When ready, salmon should be soft and easy to break apart with a fork.

Use the rest of the butter or oil on a pan and sauté spinach for a few minutes. Add salt and pepper to your liking. Serve together with salmon and enjoy

Serves 2 – 4

Pulled Pork and Afelia

. . .

*T*his is an excellent dish for any pork lovers out there. Afelia is a type of regional pork dish from Cyprus consisting of red wine and coriander seeds.

*I*ngredients

- 3 lbs. pork shoulder
- 1 whole garlic
- 2 tbsp. coriander, crushed
- 2 tsp. ground black pepper
- 2 tsp. ground cinnamon
- ½ cup olive oil
- ¾ cup red wine
- 2 red onions

*P*reparation

Slice red onions into thin pieces. Cut garlic in half. Mix all ingredients (wine, thyme, black pepper, olive oil, coriander seeds, and ground cinnamon) in a bag.

Salt the pork and place inside marinade bag, making sure you get rid of all the air in the bag then seal it. Refrigerate for at least 12 hours for best taste.

Preheat oven to 260 degrees and place the meat and marinade in oven safe container. When pouring out the marinade leave the onions with the rest of the pork. Leave inside the oven for around 5 to 6 hours. Alternatively, use a slow cooker for 8 to 12 hours.

When done, pull the pork apart with a fork and serve with your choice of sides of veggies or coleslaw

Serves 4 - 6

Pimiento Cheese Meatballs

*I*ts cheese inside meatballs. Meatballs with cheese. What else could you ask for?

*I*ngredients

- 25 oz. ground beef (lean or fatty your choice)
- 2 tbsp. butter or Ghee for frying
- 4 oz. cheddar cheese grated or your choice of cheese
- 1 tbsp. Dijon mustard
- 1/3 cup Keto mayonnaise
- 1 tsp. paprika powder form (or any other chili powder)
- ¼ cup pimiento pepper or jalapeño
- 1 pinch of cayenne pepper, ground
- 1 egg
- salt and pepper

*P*reparation

Mix all ingredients for pimiento cheese (cheese, your choice of peppers, paprika, mayonnaise, mustard, and ground cayenne). Leave this aside for a few minutes

Mix ground beef with egg into the mixture you just made. Make sure your hands are clean! Or use a large spoon to combine the ingredients into the meat and egg.

Make large meatballs out of the marinated meat (or however big you desire). Get a pan going with butter, oil, or Ghee over medium. Fry meatballs until they are cooked all the way through.

When done it is ready to serve with your choice of vegetables and homemade sauces.

Serves 2 - 4

KETO SNACK AND DESSERTS RECIPES

THE BEST KETO snacks are the ones that take minimal effort to make but leave you feeling satisfied. In a way, the Keto snack is competing against the snack food you may be used to eating. Things like Oreo cookies and peanut butter sandwiches. With low-carb, you can't have any of that stuff. And don't even think about reaching for some sugary treat. Instead, you will have to satisfy yourself by using whole foods. This may mean adding buttery sauces to vegetables as a dip or simply eating smaller portions of meat. A Keto snack doesn't have to be all one thing.

*I*ncluded in this section are some different ways to make Keto friendly dips to ramp up those calories when you need them. As with any other diet, your snacks shouldn't be too high in caloric value so be careful with what you eat. Take the time to portion out your snacks.

. . .

*K*eto desserts are kind of an oxymoron. Usually, to make something taste good you will have to use some form of sugar. This can come in the form of fructose found in fruit or by using an artificial sweetener. The way you go about making your desserts is up to you. Many Keto dessert recipes will ultimately result in a higher sugar or artificial sweetener intake. Because of this, desserts should be eaten only occasionally. Certainly not every day, and no more than three times a week.

A snack can be anything, from an apple to a bowl of berries. Shakes made from whole ingredients, juices and so on are also good options. A handful of nuts will go a far way. Snacks don't have to be involved or contrived like some other recipes. Here are some recipes for your inspiration.

Low-Carb Kohlslaw

*I*t may not look like the dish you are familiar with, but it still packs a might taste

*I*ngredient

- 15 oz. kohlrabis or your choice of cabbage, radish, and carrots
- 1 cup Keto mayonnaise
- salt and pepper
- Additional herbs like parsley and cilantro for taste

*P*reparation

Shred the veggies however fine you wish. Make sure you get rid of any extraneous roots or earthy parts on radishes and kohlrabi. Then simply add the mayo along with any other herbs for flavoring.

Serves 2 to 4

Keto Mayonnaise

*T*he low-carb version of the stuff you can buy at the store. It's not much different!

*I*ngredients

- 1 egg yolk
- 1 tsp. Dijon mustard
- 2 – 4 tsp. lemon juice (more if you wish for a zesty mayo)
- 1 tsp. water
- ¼ cup extra virgin olive oil
- ½ cup avocado oil
- Salt

*P*reparation

Put the egg yolk, mustard, lemon juice and water in a bowl and whisk until evenly distributed. Add salt at this time if you wish to. This is easier done with a mechanical whisk rather than by hand.

As you are whisking away, let a few drops of oil into the mixture. Note that you are trying to make a creamy, thick mayo and the oil will appear translucent. Make sure you whisk well enough so that the oil isn't obviously visible. Add oil on a drop-by-drop basis until mayo is sufficiently thick, at which point you can add a steady stream of oil.

When all traces of the oil are gone and the mayo looks thick and fluffy, you are done. Keep stored in the fridge.

Keto Buttercream

*B*uttercream is a sweet snack that you can eat alone or with fruit and veggies. Be careful not to indulge in too much of it though! You can also use it regularly with your bullet-proof coffee (in small dashes)

*I*ngredients

- 2 tsp. vanilla extract
- 1 -2 tsp. erythritol
- 8 oz. regular butter
- 1 ½ tsp. ground cinnamon

*P*reparation

With very low heat slightly brown ¼ of the butter in a pain. It should turn a slight amber color unless you manage to burn it.

With the browned butter mix into a small bowl and add the rest of the uncooked butter in. Whisk by hand or with a mechanical whisk if preferred until mixture is fluffy.

Add cinnamon and erythritol for extra taste. Erythritol is an alternative sweetener, it is up to you if you want to use it.

Buffalo Drumsticks with Chili Aioli

*A*ioli is a type of Mediterranean sauce typically made using garlic and olive oil. It makes an excellent side for many a drumstick!

*I*ngredients

- 2 lbs. chicken drumstick
- 2 tbsp. white vinegar
- 1 tbsp. tomato paste
- 1 tbsp. Tabasco
- 2 tbsp. paprika
- 1 tsp. salt
- butter or olive oil for baking dish
- 1 garlic clove minced
- 2/3 cup Keto mayonnaise

*P*reparation

Marinade drumsticks using a plastic bag. Add in vinegar, tomato paste, Tabasco, and paprika powder. Let marinade for around 30 minutes or longer if left in the fridge.

Preheat oven to 450 degrees. Get a baking dish ready with your choice of oil and put drumsticks on it. Bake for 30 to 45 minutes (drumsticks should get a reddish brown color)

Mix mayonnaise, garlic, and paprika chili power together. Use as a dip and enjoy

Serves 4 – 6

Herb Butter

A fluffy, creamy lemony butter. For use with all your favorite snacks and even as a side for the main course dinner

*I*ngredients

- 1 garlic clove pressed by hand or machine
- 1 tsp. lemon juice
- ½ tbsp. garlic powder
- 4 tbsp. finely chopped parsley
- 5 oz. butter or Ghee at room temp
- Salt and pepper

*P*reparation

Put all ingredients in a bowl and mix until everything is well distributed. Let sit for around 15 minutes for flavor to set. Store any leftovers in the refrigerator. That's it!

Spinach Dip

. . .

*I*ts spinach as a dip. Combines the flavor of your favorite leafy green with fatty goodness. A Keto favorite. Use as a dip for your snacks or as a sauce

*I*ngredients

- 1 cup Keto mayonnaise
- 2 tsp. lemon juice
- 4 tbsp. sour cream
- ¼ tsp. ground black pepper
- 1 tsp. onion powder
- 2 tbsp. olive oil
- 2 tbsp. parsley
- 2 oz. frozen baby spinach
- 1 tbsp. dill
- ½ tsp. salt

*P*reparation

That or warm up frozen spinach in the microwave. Make sure the spinach is as dry as possible. Either dry them off or wait for it to evaporate.

Mix all ingredients (including spinach) in a bowl. Give at least 10 minutes for flavors to set. Ready to serve after that! Keep refrigerated

Cilantro Butter

. . .

ou either love or hate cilantro. If you are part of the cilantro camp, you will thoroughly enjoy this fluffy butter

Ingredients

- ¼ tsp. ground black pepper
- 1 tbsp. lime juice
- 5 oz. regular butter
- ½ cup chopped cilantro
- 2 tbsp. extra virgin olive oil
- t tsp. salt
- ½ tsp. coriander ground

Preparation

Use an immersion blender to mix oil and cilantro. You could also do it by hand but this may be trickier. Then get your butter, salt, ground coriander, ground pepper, and lime juice and add them into the mix. Mix thoroughly until evenly distributed and allow a few minutes for flavors to set.

Keep refrigerated

Easy Chicken Fritters

he closest you can get to eating chicken nuggets on an all-clean Keto diet. If you have a food processor or blender, you can make these in a jiffy.

. . .

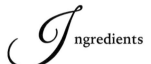

Ingredients

- 2 large eggs
- 3 celery stalk
- 1 tsp. dried oregano
- 13 oz. boneless chicken thighs (or breast)
- ¾ cup fine coconut flour
- 1 cup coconut oil, avocado oil, extra virgin olive oil or Ghee
- 1 tsp. cumin ground finely

Preparation

First make the marinade by throwing in the seasonings, chopped celery, and onion into a food processor or powerful blender. Put it on high until everything is evenly and finely minced. Add your raw eggs and chicken into the food processor and put it on high again until you have a thick looking paste.

Get a large skilling going with medium heat. Add your choice of oil and let heat for a little while.

With the coconut flour scoop two tablespoons of the paste, shape it into a ball, and put into the flour. It is easier to use a bowl full of flower and dump them in there. Turn the ball of paste over to fully cover with coconut flour. Toss each ball around your hands until the flour has settled evenly. Do this for all of the paste.

Once the oil is sizzling, add fritters for frying. Do some in small batches, depending on the size of the skillet. They should not touch. Allow each to fry for about 3 minutes. Remove them carefully with a spoon or tongs. Make sure to dry off excess oil with a paper towel. These can be eaten right away. Enjoy with your choice of homemade dip.

Serves 4 – 6

Chocolate and Macadamia Nut Fat Bomb

a fat bomb, as you will soon learn, is the preferred dessert for many Keto practitioners. Still, don't go too crazy with these. The best part? No baking required!

*I*ngredients

- 1 tbsp. MCT oil
- ¼ cup sugar-free dark chocolate alternatively sweetened chocolate chips
- 1 ½ oz. raw macadamia nut
- Sea salt

*P*reparation

Melt chocolate chips for 50 seconds inside the microwave. Use microwave safe bowl. You want them soft enough so that you can easily stir them. Pour MCT oil into the blend along with a pinch of sea salt and mix thoroughly.

Get a truffle or chocolate mold and place 3 macadamia nut pieces per mold. Add chocolate mixture to each mold making sure nuts are covered all the way.

Put molds in freezer until chocolate is solid (usually takes about 30 minutes to an hour depending on freezer settings)

Low-Carb Lemon Ice Cream

*W*ho says you can't have ice cream on the Keto diet? Require ice cream maker or a bit of ingenuity

*I*ngredients

- 3 eggs
- ¼ tsp. yellow food coloring (for appearance but not needed)
- 1/3 cup erythritol or other alternative sweeteners
- 1 lemon for zest and juice
- 1 ¾ heavy whipping cream

*P*reparation

Wash the lemon and grate the zest from peel. Try not to get too much of the actual lemon. Squeeze the juice out in a separate container and leave alone for now.

Separate and beat egg whites. Meanwhile, whisk the yolks in with sweetener of choice until fluffy. Then add lemon juice and a little bit of food coloring if desired. Then put egg whites into your yolk.

Whip the cream until fluffy in a separate bowl and then add the egg and yolk mix.

Use your preferred ice cream to process the mixture and freeze accordingly.

Alternatively, put the bowl in the freezer and stir every half hour, making sure it doesn't stay frozen. If it does freeze, let it thaw outside for a little before stirring again.

Vanilla Custard

*K*eto custard—now without dairy!

*I*ngredients

- 1 tsp. erythritol or your choice of alternative sweetener. Optional for added taste
- 6 egg yolk
- ¼ cup melted coconut oil or regular butter
- 1 tsp. vanilla extract
- ½ cup unsweetened almond milk

*P*reparation

In a medium bowl whisk the egg yolk, vanilla extract, milk, and sweetener if so desired.

After those ingredients are evenly distributed mix in melted oil or butter. Ensure that oil isn't piping hot. It just needs to be a little warm.

Now simmer a little bit of water on a saucepan and place contents of the bowl into the pan. Continue to whisk mixture until it is nice and fluffy. If you have a thermometer ready, you want the heat to be at 140 degrees. Takes about 5 minutes to cook. Store egg whites for later.

Can either be served warm or chilled.

4 to 6 servings

Hot Chocolate

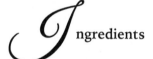 fine addition to your bulletproof coffee, all Keto.

Ingredients

- ¼ tsp. vanilla extract
- 1 cup boiling water
- 1 tbsp. cocoa powder
- 1 oz. regular butter
- 1 tsp. erythritol or your choice of alternative sweetener if so desired

Preparation

Put all ingredients together into an immersion blender. Alternatively, mix each ingredient one by one into boiling water (but it's not very efficient by hand). There should be a thin foam when done.

Ready to enjoy as is, piping hot.

Pumpkin Spice Latte

. . .

*F*or those who are all about pumpkin spice

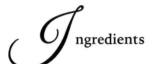

*I*ngredients

- 1 cup boiling water
- 1 – 2 tsp. instant coffee
- 1 oz. regular butter
- 1 tsp. pumpkin pie spice

*P*reparation

Get ingredients (spices, coffee powder, and butter) into immersion blender. You can also mix them with a regular blender if you don't have an immersion blender. Don't actually mix yet though.

Add the boiling water to the mixed powders and now blend. Should be foamy at the top.

Ready to serve with cinnamon, whipped cream, or even more pumpkin spice.

15 DAY KETOGENIC DIET MEAL PLAN

THE PERFECT KETO meal plan is one that is simple, hits your macros, and respects your carbohydrate limits. But designing such a plan can be difficult. Keep in mind that the recipes and food suggestions provided are merely suggestions. You can replace ingredients, add ingredients, and alter portion sizes as desired. Keto success thrives on staying as low-carb as possible. What foods you decide to eat are largely up to you, keeping in mind their carbohydrate contents. Snack and desserts tend to be higher in carbs, so eat these in moderation and never in large portions.

Take advantage of leftovers wherever possible. Heat them up the next day as a main course or as a snack. Repurpose the ingredients to make another dish. Never throw away food or let it sit in the fridge to the point where you must throw it away. Make things easier on yourself wherever possible. If this means staying up the night before preparing some of your meals then so be it. Many of the recipes provided have multiple servings. These are ideal for eating throughout the week instead of having to cook another whole meal.

*N*obody likes to take time out of their busy days to prepare all of their meals. Some meals will be more involved than others. This is why the meal plan uses the recipes included in this book as well as self-explanatory lunch and dinner platters that don't require instructions. These are as simple as getting a large plastic container and filling it up with your choice of meat, side of nuts, and side of veggies with mayo or some other sauce for a dip. Such meals are easy to make but still enough to keep you satisfied.

*D*ay One

Breakfast – Easy Breakfast Platter with bacon, hard-boiled eggs, and avocados. Your choice of sauce, and or a cup of sautéed leafy greens

Lunch – Sirloin steak salad

Afternoon snack – a handful of raw almonds

Dinner – Fried Salmon with broccoli in lemon mayo

Snack before bed – Banana

*D*ay Two

Breakfast – Guacamole breakfast stack

Lunch – Leftover sirloin steak salad

Snack – Baby carrot platter with a side of herb butter

Dinner – Pork chops with green beans and avocado

Snack before bed – a handful of raw almonds

Day Three

Breakfast – 16 oz. smoothie of berries and almond milk (use the unsweetened kind for fewer carbs)

Lunch – Cauliflower mac and cheese

Afternoon snack – half a medium apple

Dinner – Leftover salmon or pork chops. Also, sauté another batch of leafy greens or broccoli

Snack before bed – Small bowl of vanilla custard

Day Four

Breakfast – Cauliflower breakfast toast with your choice of greens and dip

Lunch – Lemon butter chicken with your choice of 1-cup leafy greens as a side (more if desired)

Afternoon snack – Two buffalo drumsticks with a side of aioli or your choice of dip

Dinner – Sausage Alfredo with zucchini noodles

Snack before bed – 2 string kinds of cheese

. . .

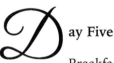

Day Five

Breakfast – Mushroom omelet

Lunch – leftover lemon butter chicken with your choice of leafy greens

Afternoon snack – two or three hard-boiled eggs with a side of baby carrots

Dinner – leftover sausage Alfredo

Snack before bed – 2 or 3 macadamia fat bombs

Day Six

Breakfast – Breakfast Tuna Platter

Lunch – Cheese and steak filled peppers

Afternoon snack – Kale chips, roasted

Dinner – Cabbage needle beef stroganoff

Snack before bed – a handful of almonds with a small helping of your choice of cheese

Day Seven

Breakfast – Easy Breakfast Platter with bacon, hard-boiled eggs, and avocados. Your choice of sauce, and or a cup of sautéed leafy greens

Lunch – leftover cheese and steak filled peppers

Afternoon snack – 20 – 30 all natural olives

Dinner – leftover beef stroganoff

Snack before bed – 2 or 3 macadamia fat bombs

*D*ay Eight

Breakfast – 3 scrambled eggs, Mexican style with diced onion, tomato, green pepper, and optional jalapeño. Your choice side of 1 cup leafy greens or veggies sautéed in olive oil

Lunch – Sirloin steak salad

Afternoon snack – 3 – 5 chicken fritters

Dinner – low-carb traditional beef stew

Snack before bed – Keto Hot chocolate

*D*ay Nine

Breakfast – Mushroom omelet

Lunch – leftover sirloin steak

Afternoon snack – pumpkin spice latte

Dinner – leftover traditional beef stew

Snack before bed – a handful of coconut meat (about 40g)

*D*ay Ten

Breakfast – Guacamole breakfast stack

Lunch – Lemon butter chicken with your choice 1 – 2 cup side of vegetables or leafy greens

Afternoon snack – 50g avocado (about half medium-sized avocado)

Dinner – pimiento cheese meatballs with your choice 1 – 2 cup side of vegetables or leafy greens

Snack before bed – small bowl of vanilla custard

*D*ay Eleven

Breakfast – 16 oz. berry and almond milkshake

Lunch – leftover pimiento cheese meatballs and side of veggies

Afternoon snack – leftover lemon butter chicken with spinach dip

Dinner – pulled pork with afelia, side of veggies, and your choice side of cheese

Snack before bed: 2 string cheese

*D*ay Twelve

Breakfast – Cauliflower breakfast toast with your choice of veggies and dip

Lunch – 5 to 8 chicken fritters with your choice 1 – 2 cups of veggies or leafy greens

Afternoon snack – a handful of almonds and side of cheese

Dinner – leftover pulled pork

Snack before bed – Keto lemon ice cream

• • •

Day Thirteen

Breakfast – Three boiled eggs with a side of asparagus and Keto mayonnaise

Lunch – Cauliflower mac and cheese

Afternoon snack – 20 to 30 raw pistachios

Dinner – Pesto salmon with spinach

Snack before bed – 2 to 3 macadamia nut fat bombs

Day Fourteen

Breakfast – Breakfast tuna platter

Lunch – Sirloin steak salad

Afternoon snack – sliced fruit platter of kiwi, strawberry, and blueberries with a side of Keto buttercream

Dinner – leftover Pesto Salmon. Make another batch of spinach or your choice leafy greens

Snack before bed – banana

Day Fifteen

Breakfast – Easy Breakfast Platter with bacon, hard-boiled eggs, and avocados. Your choice of sauce, and or a cup of sautéed leafy greens

Lunch – leftover sirloin steak with a side of cilantro butter

ELYSE BOSE

Afternoon snack – 2 hardboiled eggs, side of baby carrots

Dinner – Pork cup with green beans and avocado

CONCLUSION

This concludes the content for *Keto Diet for beginners*. You should have learned the basics of Keto, how it works, and what the justifications for it are. You should have also gotten the general feel for how to cook meals the Keto way. Remember to emphasize the role of healthy fats, veggies, and especially animal proteins. The recipes used in this book lean towards the specialty side of things—they require more ingredients than you would typically find in your cupboard. All of the major ingredients mentioned here, like salmon, pork and chicken are universal to most households. You can whip up a quick Keto meal simply having the bare essentials, which are some fatty oil or butter, meat, and some leafy greens. As always, have some salt and pepper handy—both for taste and sodium needs.

The 15-day meal plan is open to suggestions from you. If you cook for a family or a group of people you are less likely to have leftovers throughout the week, for example. You may be allergic to dairy and can't consume cheese. Make changes wherever you see fit and feel free to look up additional recipes online. Don't feel like you have to stick with the meal plan exactly as it is written, or that you need to eat snacks in between. Ramping up the portion sizes it is possible to avoid snacking altogether.

Who knows, maybe you will make the permanent switch to Keto in time. Whether for weight loss, to treat diabetes or simply to live a healthier lifestyle away from sugary and refined foods. The only people who lose out are the food companies that still market these products regularly. You are by no means obligated to follow along with them.

As a final note, never feel that you must sacrifice taste for health. A diet doesn't mean bland food. We aren't eating saltine crackers with cold cucumber soup here. We are eating protein-rich whole foods, veggies, and healthy fats. Maybe the taste isn't as good as sugar (most of us are addicted to that stuff) but in time you will forget all about sweet tasting things. Bring on the flank steak and pork chops, please.

INTERMITTENT FASTING

Accelerate Weight Loss, Reset Your Metabolism - Keto Diet Recipes Included

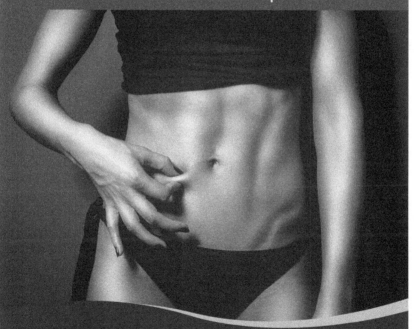

Elyse Bose

INTRODUCTION

Congratulations on downloading your personal copy of *Intermittent Fasting,* and thank you for doing so. I have provided you with many ways to drop the pounds using the intermittent fasting techniques and your ketogenic diet recipes. First, let's see what the plan involves for your future.

Intermittent Fasting is not so much a diet as it is a way of life. It allows you to eat what you want when you want – within the Keto-genic diet plan. However, use caution when eating what you want when you want because it can have harmful effects on your health. The idea behind fasting is to clear the body of toxins and harmful elements, which is slowing you down and causing you to carry excessive weight.

So, when we say you can eat what you want when you want, you still have to make healthy balanced choices. On your fasting plan, you should only eat when you are hungry and at a predetermined time, but even then, ask yourself if you are *really* hungry or is it something else such as boredom.

It's been observed that in short periods of time, fasting can speed up the healing process and permit the body to recover from serious diseases. Some conditions and diseases such as arthritis and lupus, persistent skin conditions like psoriasis and eczema, as well as Crohn's disease and ulcerative colitis have been gotten rid of and/or cleared up. In addition, conditions such as angina and high blood pressure are quickly eliminated. In most situations, these cases were long-lasting if not permanent.

Fasting has been around for thousands of years. It has its roots in various religions. What purpose did fasting serve under those circumstances? How is fasting done with modern-day religions? Can fasting be done for non-religious reasons?

Why has fasting become such a trend in recent years? What is it about fasting that is causing so many people to see substantial weight loss and improved overall health?

There is so much information out there about fasting and intermittent fasting that people can get lost in the information and possibly end up hurting themselves if they are not diligent and careful.

Other things to think about as we begin learning more about fasting are some of the myths and misinformation that is out there. Let's begin!

INTERMITTENT FASTING BASICS
INTRODUCTION

TYPES of Intermittent Fasting

*J*f you are interested in trying out the benefits of intermittent fasting for yourself, but you have an irregular schedule or are not sure if it is for you, then skipping a meal or two now and then maybe the type of intermittent fasting for you. Getting into a fasting routine is vital to see the maximum results for your effort, but that doesn't occasionally mean that fasting doesn't come with some benefits as well.

What's more, once you have tried skipping a meal now and then, you can see for yourself just how easy it is, which in turn can lead to more positive changes down the line. With so many intermittent fasting options available the odds are good that one fits your schedule, so give it a try. What have you got to lose (besides a few pounds)?

The 16/8 Method

When searching the internet for information on Leangains, it takes extraordinarily little effort to find Martin Berkhan. He's a model, nutritional consultant, and personal trainer. He has made the 16/8 or Leangains Diet popular.

The technique involves fasting for either 16 hours for men or 14 hours for women before allowing yourself to consume a reasonable amount of calories for the remaining 8 to 10 hours. During this period, you should only consume things that have zero calories including black coffee (a splash of cream is fine), water, diet soda, and sugar-free gum. The easiest way to attempt this schedule is to stop eating after dinner in the evening and wait 14 or 16 hours from there. This means skipping breakfast and eating again in the early afternoon.

Again, the specifics of when you fast are not nearly as important as ensuring that you fast for the same period of time as regularly as possible. If you vary your fasting period too much, it can lead to an erratic change in your hormones which among other things can make it much more difficult for your body to shed any excess weight.

If you find yourself without the time required to eat a proper meal to break your fast normally, you should at least eat some-thing to keep your body on the correct cycle. If you are exercising as well as intermittently fasting it is important to ensure that you are eating more carbohydrates than fats while you are working out while on days you are not exercising the opposite is true. It is also important to ensure that you keep your protein intake at a steady level and stay away from processed foods whenever possible.

The benefits of this type of fasting are that it is extremely flexible so that it will work for a wide variety of schedules. Most people find it helpful to either eat two large meals during the 8 or 10-hour period feeding period or split that time into three smaller meals as that is the way most people are already programmed.

On days you are exercising as well as fasting it is important to attempt to and always break your fast with a mix of protein, veggies, and fruit. If you generally go to the gym directly after you have broken your fast, it is important to include enough carbohydrates to give your muscles the energy they need to get the most out of your workout.

If you are planning to exercise, it is generally best to start the early afternoon off right with a medium calorie meal. Then exercise within three hours before eating a larger meal soon afterward. In this larger meal, it is important to add a larger portion of complex carbohydrates, and you can even have a little dessert as long as it is in moderation. Remember, fasting is different than dieting.

On the days you do not plan on exercising, it is important to adjust your caloric intake appropriately. Start by limiting your carbohydrate intake and instead focus on eating lots of protein, dark green, leafy vegetables, and fruit in moderation. Unlike on days you are exercising the first meal you eat on rest days should be your largest in terms of caloric intake with this one meal counting for about 40 percent of your daily total.

Remember, during this meal you should be taking in more protein than anything else. For your final meal during rest days, it is important to include a protein source that will take lots of time to digest which in turn means it will keep you full for more of your fast the following morning. It also provides the body with enough stored amino acids to prevent it from breaking down muscle during the fast.

The 5:2 or Fast Diet

For women, just restrict calories for two days weekly by having 2 meals (250 calories each). Men can have 600 calories or 300 calories for 2 meals. The rule-of-thumb is based on men needing 2,400 calories and women 2,000 calories. Eat as you usually do on the remainder of the week using the ketogenic diet plan. There are not that many statistics on this diet for women, but it is considered safe. Consider consuming about 1/4 of your regular calorie intake.

Soups are an excellent choice for your fasting days. These are several other examples:

- Baked or boiled eggs
- Natural yogurt and berries
- Tea
- Black coffee
- Plenty of water
- Generous portions of veggies
- Lean meat or grilled fish
- Cauliflower rice

The Warrior Diet

The Warrior Diet takes the 16/8 program and kicks it up a notch by suggesting that you fast for roughly 20 hours out of each day followed by one meal where you get all of your calories in the four remaining hours of the day. This form of intermittent fasting follows the belief that humans are naturally nocturnal eaters.

Therefore, eating at night helps the body easily process the nutri- ·
ents it needs. In this case, fasting is a bit of a misnomer as during the 20-hour period you are allowed to eat a serving of raw vegetables or fruits and maybe a serving of protein if you just can't otherwise continue.

This works because it causes the body's natural sympathetic nervous system to activate a flight or fight response which in turns

INTERMITTENT FASTING

increases your natural levels of alertness, and increases energy while at the same time increasing the amount of fat burned. The large meal each evening then allows the body to focus on repairing itself and improving its muscles. When following the Warrior Diet, it's important to start your evening meal with veggies, followed by protein, fat, and carbohydrates.

This form of fasting is popular for two reasons. First, the fact that a few small and reasonable snacks are allowed during the fasting process which makes this type of fasting attractive to those who are attempting the practice for the first time. Second, nearly everyone who attempts this form of fasting reports a significant amount of increased energy throughout the day, as well as an increase in the amount of fat lost per week.

On the other hand, the relatively strict nature of this diet can make it difficult for some people to follow for long periods of time. The timing of the large meal can also make it difficult for some people to follow because of the way it naturally interferes with some social engagements. Finally, some people simply don't like having to eat their food in a specific order, try it for yourself and see what works for you.

Alternate Day Diet

This form of intermittent fasting actually means you never have to go long without food if you so choose. Every other day you should eat regularly, and on the off-days, you merely consume one-fifth of the calories you usually intake on the average days.

The average daily caloric consumption is between 2,000 and 2,500 calories which means that the regular off-day varies between 400 and 500 calories. If you enjoy exercising every day, then this form of intermittent fasting may not be for you since you will have to limit your workouts on off-days severely.

91

When you first start this form of intermittent fasting, the easiest way to make it through the low-calorie days is by trying a variety of protein shakes. It's important to work back to natural foods on these days because they will always be healthier than the shakes.

This form of intermittent fasting is all about losing weight. Those who try it tend to average between two and three pounds lost per week. If you attempt the Alternate Day Diet, it is critical to eat regularly on your full-calorie days. Binging will not only negate any progress you have made, but it can also cause severe damage to your body if continued over time.

Crescendo Method

This is a method that is ranked as one suitable for women since you can begin fasting without irritating your hormones or shocking any part of your body using this technique. This is one of the safest programs for women which utilize a fasting window of 12-16 hours. You can enjoy your meals for 8-12 hours. Space it out for a few days such as Monday, Wednesday, and Friday. If you have failed other diets, this might be your answer. After a two-week time period, add one more day of active fasting to your schedule.

Clearing Up Intermittent Fasting Misconceptions

Misconception 1: Fasting Causes the Body to go into Starvation Mode

Starvation is not controlled; there is no discernable end to the lack of food, and it is not voluntary. When you think about the number of meals you eat over the course of a year (let's stick to the three meals a day), is it really possible for the body to go into starvation mode, if it misses just one meal during that time? That's over 1,000 meals during the year, 1, 095 to be exact. Even if the body missed those 95 meals during the year, how likely is it that the body would go into starvation mode? It just wouldn't happen.

Remember, starvation doesn't have a determined end to being without food; it doesn't know when the next meal is going to come. Fasting has a meal at the end of it, whether it's three hours or three days later.

Misconception 2: Fasting Can Lead To Overeating

This is simply not true. For instance, let's say that after a 24-hour fast, a person consumes a total of 2,834 calories, but normally would have eaten about 2,325 calories. That is an increase of only 509 calories. Now, if that same person had eaten normally over the same two-day period, they would have consumed 5,668 calories.

The difference between eating 5,668 calories over two days and only a 509-calorie increase over the same two days becomes insignificant. In fact, some have observed over time, as the fasting continues, their appetites seem to decrease.

Misconception 3: Low Blood Sugar is caused by Fasting

When your blood sugar gets low, it can lead to shaking and sweating. However, the body has tight control of blood sugar regulation. When fasting, the body breaks down something called glycogen, which is stored in the liver for a short period of time. We experience this at night when we sleep, and this helps keep your blood sugar levels normal during the night-time fasting period.

Now, if you fast for periods longer than 36 hours, this glycogen becomes depleted, and the liver can now manufacture new glucose. The liver does this through an amazing process called gluconeogenesis. As a result, the process of breaking down fat produces a by-product called glycerol.

Related to this myth is that the only energy that brain cells can use is glucose. Not true! The brain can also use ketones as an energy source. When fat is metabolized, it produces little particles called ketones. When food is not readily obtainable, we survive and function well because ketones are the main provider of the energy we need to get through that period.

Intermittent Fasting Concerns

Heartburn: If you have chosen a plan where you have larger meals, you may need to try another fasting method to remedy the issue. Once a fast cycle is completed, you also tend to want to eat faster. Eat slowly and avoid lying down right after a meal or for a minimum of 30 minutes.

Headaches: As you enter ketosis, you may experience headaches. Add some extra salt to your diet to help diminish the issue. It will go away.

*M*uscle Cramps: You could be experiencing low magnesium levels. Try a supplement over-the-counter and soak in some Epsom salts. Just add one cup to your bath water. Soak for about 30 minutes for the magnesium salts to absorb through your skin.

Other Risk Factors of Intermittent Fasting

- If you are taking prescription medications, you can have issues on taking them on an empty stomach. If you have diabetes, Metformin may cause diarrhea or nausea. Iron supplements may also cause stomach discomfort. Aspirin may also cause an upset stomach or possible ulcers.

- People who are underweight (BMI≤ 18.5) are malnourished or have other known nutrient deficiencies

- Children under 18 need more nutrients to grow.

- Individuals with diabetes mellitus – type 1 or type 2

- Individuals who experience many times a drop in his/her blood sugar levels

Intermittent Fasting & Exercise

You should work out while fasting. If you're just beginning to fast, it might be advisable to hold off on your vigorous workouts for a couple of weeks and do something lighter until you are used to fasting, especially if you are used to eating before your workouts.

The benefits of working out in a fasted state are tremendous. According to Jerome H., "You become more sensitive to insulin and allow the human growth hormone to help you burn fat and build muscle."

In short, if you work out in a fasted state, the body will turn to the existing fat stores to burn for energy instead of using the food you ate before your workout for that energy. As a result, your body becomes more efficient at burning its existing fat. Your body will still rely on stored body fat to burn for energy, whether you want a 'rippled' body or just want to be slimmer and fit into your clothes better.

There is no consensus about when to work out while fasting, except considering when your first meal for the day will be. As we've mentioned, fasting is completely flexible. So, if you are eating breakfast in the morning and fasting for the rest of the day and overnight, then consider working out before breakfast.

However, if your meals are later in the day, consider working out about an hour before that meal, whether it's around noon or even later. With the 16/8, you have a window of eight hours that you can eat. The idea is to work out in a fasted state, so make sure your workout before your first meal, whatever time that might be.

If you are just getting acquainted with fasting, take it easy; get used to fasting first, for about a week or even two. Then, slowly add exercise back into your routine. Start with a brisk walk and slowly work up to running. Next, add in an interval of weight training.

Above all else, always listen to your body. If something doesn't feel right, then stop and talk to your doctor. Make sure you speak to him/her before starting any new exercise program.

Intermittent Fasting Tips for Success

Make Sure You Maintain A Calorie Deficit: While this is true for any diet, it is especially true for intermittent fasting as it can be especially easy to overeat once you do eat in such a way that it negates any benefits you might have felt.

Remember To Remain Consistent: Regardless of the type of weight loss technique that you choose to pursue, it is important to choose one and stick with it. Attempting an intermittent fast for a few days before switching to the paleo diet before trying out a low-carb approach will only cause your body to freak out and hold on to every possible calorie until it figures out what in the world is happening.

*R*emember, fasting regularly and consistently is the surest way to see any of its benefits. Only after your body has time to adjust to your new routine will it then be able to adapt appropriately and begin to increase the number of positive enzymes and neural pathways to maximize weight loss using this method. Consider consistency the ace-in-the-hole of proactive weight loss success.

Maintain Self-Control: Intermittent fasting only works if your body goes completely without food for at least twelve hours. Any caloric intake resets the cycle. As such, it is extremely important to ensure that you maintain control of your bodily urges if you hope to see real results from this type of approach. Remember, fasting for at least twelve hours only allows you to each normally or slightly more than an average meal, it does not give you a license to eat everything in sight. Keeping your appetite in check is a strict requirement for success.

INTERMITTENT FASTING & THE KETO DIET

YOU NEED to make sure that you derive as much nutrition as possible from the foods you eat during your fasting. You should eat foods prepared using the ketogenic diet techniques, including satisfying meals laden with veggies, animal proteins, and berries.

Healthy Carbohydrates: You already have a very good idea of what healthy carbs are since you will be using the ketogenic diet plan, including sweet potatoes, legumes, and fruit.

Shellfish & Fish: The American Heart Association recommends you eat a minimum of two servings every week. You can enjoy 3.5 oz. for each serving by using canned light tuna or Alaskan salmon. Make a sandwich or save the carbs and have a salad.

Pork: Serve and enjoy pork tenderloin, sirloin, and loin chops which are very lean cuts of pork. Prepare 3-ounce servings to get 23 grams of protein and your B vitamins.

Skinless Chicken or Turkey: Choose the leanest cut of white meat you can find for about 25 grams of protein, B vitamins, and selenium.

90% Or Leaner Ground Beef: Get your protein, iron, zinc, and 22 grams of protein with just 3 oz. of lean beef.

Eggs: Consider eggs at just 6 grams of protein for one egg. Most of the protein is in the egg white. You can also choose a hard-boiled egg as a snack or in with a salad.

Beans & Lentils: Eat many of these as possible. Each half a cup it is only 9 grams. They are a good source of folate, fiber, and iron.

Transitioning To the Keto Diet

*A*s you begin your intermittent fasting techniques using the ketogenic diet, you will need to distinguish between physical hunger and psychological hunger.

If you are experiencing physical hunger, you will gradually have the urge, and it can be postponed. Any type of food will satisfy your hunger, and you will be calm when you stop eating. After you suppress your physical hunger, you will be satisfied, not guilty.

Emotional hunger is a little bit different since you feel urgent or anxious and it comes on suddenly. You're craving specific foods which can include ice cream, chocolate, or any other trigger food that you enjoy. After you have finished eating, you will also feel annoyed with yourself or guilty about what you have eaten and how much you have eaten. There is 'the evidence' that you needed to hear; it is emotional hunger!

*P*repare A Menu & Food Plan: You will be surprised how many tasty items you can enjoy that are full of healthy nutrients. Be sure to properly calculate the macronutrients of each recipe you prepare for your daily meal plan.

5-Day Plan: Step-By-Step To Intermittent Fasting:

*U*se this as a guideline, so you have a better understanding of how to easily change over from your regular dieting habits to a much cleaner way of eating using the ketogenic plan and fasting.

Day 1: Don't Eat After Dinner:

*Y*ou'll get hungry around 8 or 9 o'clock, so try one of these ways to get through the evening hours before bedtime:

- Prepare a warm cup of tea or a large glass of water versus a heavier food item.
- Use a minty toothpaste. Your mind will focus on this as a barrier to keep you from eating.
- If all else fails, just go to bed!

Day 2: Hold Off On The "Break-Fast" Meal:

*F*or the best results of the day, postpone your meal and prepare for a 12-hour fast.

For example, if you had your last meal at 6 pm. It is okay to have breakfast at 6 am. But, don't eat until you're hungry! Eat when it is convenient. Have a calorie-free beverage such as tea, coffee, or water.

If you work outside of your home, wait until about 10 am and eat your breakfast meal after your early morning schedule is completed.

Everyone else aims for 12 noon as the time to eat, but forego the meal if you aren't hungry. Ignore the clock; you just had breakfast, so have another glass of water.

Everyone else is having a 2 pm snack. Now, it's time for your lunch since you are probably hungry.

See how simple that was! Have dinner at 6 pm. Continue the process in the previous steps and don't eat after your evening meal – until 10 am tomorrow.

*D*ay 3: Forget Snack Time:

*Y*ou just did a 15- to 16-hour fast! It is now time to celebrate!

After lunch, do not eat until dinner. These are a few tips to help avoid snacking:

If you are a habitual snacker in the afternoon, have some more non-calorie beverages. Stay busy once you leave work. Go for a walk or call a friend.

Have dinner - regular time - 7 pm. Continue and do not have anything after dinner (until 10 am.).

Day 4: Skip The Breakfast Meal:

. . .

*T*t's really time to celebrate now. You have done another 15-hour fast, and you didn't have a snack! You had dinner at 7 pm last night and stopped eating till now without any snacks! Now, you delayed again until 10 a.m. this morning. Go ahead one more time, skip breakfast today by waiting one more hour to before you eat. This will make lunchtime your first meal of the day at 11 am.

Continue to use mindful eating and try not to eat while doing other activities.

Remember, you may just be thirsty, not hungry. Have dinner at 7 pm. Once again, do not eat after dinner, skip breakfast, don't snack in between lunch and dinner.

Day 5: Continue Moving Forward:

*T*oday, just repeat the steps. Congrats to you! You just completed a 16-hour fast.

You had dinner at 7 pm, and you skip breakfast by eating your first meal at 11 am, did not snack, and denied it again until 7 pm.

It remains easy as that. Just select your personal preference of meal times and go with the keto diet recipes and fasting.

BREAKFAST & BRUNCH CHOICES

BACON & Asparagus Muffins

*S*ervings: 12 (3 muffins each)

Total Macro Nutrients:

- 3 g Net Carbs
- 19 g Total Protein
- 41 g Total Fats
- 460 Calories

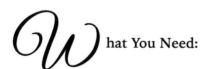hat You Need:

- Bacon slices (4 diced)
- Eggs (8 whisked)

- Asparagus spears (1 cup chopped - 7-8 spears)
- Chopped onions (2 tbsp.)
- Pepper and salt (as desired)
- Canned coconut milk (.5 cup)
- Also Needed: 12-count mini quiche cups

How To Prepare:

1. Heat up the oven until it reaches 350° Fahrenheit.
2. Cook the bacon in a frying pan. Drain on a towel. Dice when cooled.
3. Combine all of the fixings and pour into the baking tin.
4. Bake until the center is set or about 25 to 30 minutes.

Bacon Egg & Cheese Cups

Servings: 6

Total Macro Nutrients:

- 1 g Net Carbs
- 8 g Total Protein
- 7 g Total Fats
- 101 Calories

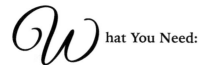 hat You Need:

- Bacon (6 strips)
- Large eggs (6)
- Cheese (.25 cup)
- Fresh spinach (1 handful)
- Pepper & Salt (as desired)

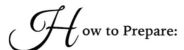 ow to Prepare:

1. Set the oven setting to 400° Fahrenheit.
2. Prepare the bacon using medium heat on the stovetop. Place on towels to drain.
3. Grease six muffin tins with a spritz of oil. Line each tin with a slice of bacon, pressing tightly to make a secure well for the eggs.
4. Drain and dry the spinach with a paper towel. Whisk the eggs and combine with the spinach.
5. Add the mixture to the prepared tins and sprinkle with cheese. Sprinkle with salt and pepper until it's like you like it.
6. Bake for 15 minutes. Remove when done and serve or cool to store in the fridge.

Bacon Hash

ervings: 2

Total Macro Nutrients:

ELYSE BOSE

- 9 g Net Carbs
- 23 g Total Protein
- 24 g Total Fats
- 366 Calories

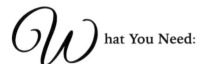 hat You Need:

- Small green pepper (1)
- Jalapenos (2)
- Small onion (1)
- Eggs (4)
- Bacon slices (6)

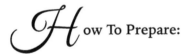 ow To Prepare:

1. Chop the bacon into chunks using a food processor. Set aside for now.
2. Slice the peppers and onions into thin strips and dice the jalapenos as small as possible.
3. Warm up a skillet and fry the veggies.
4. Once browned, combine the fixings and cook until crispy. Place on a serving dish with the eggs.

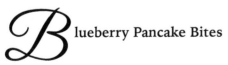 lueberry Pancake Bites

. . .

*S*ervings: 24 bites

Total Macro Nutrients:

- 7.5 g Net Carbs
- 6 g Total Protein
- 13 g Total Fats
- 188 Calories

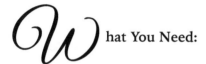hat You Need:

- Baking powder (1 tsp.)
- Water (.33 - .5 cup)
- Melted ghee (.25 cup)
- Coconut flour (.5 cup)
- Cinnamon (.5 tsp.)
- Salt (.5 tsp.)
- Eggs (4
- Vanilla extract (.5 tsp.)
- Frozen blueberries (.5 cup)
- Also Needed: Muffin tray

*H*ow to Prepare:

1. Warm up the oven to reach 325° Fahrenheit. Use a spritz of coconut oil spray to grease 24 muffin cups.
2. Combine the eggs, sweetener, and vanilla, mixing until smooth. Fold in the flour, melted ghee, salt, baking powder, and cinnamon. Stir in .33 cup of water to finish the batter.
3. The mixture should be thick. Next, divide the batter into the prepared cups with several berries in each one.
4. Bake until set (20-25 min.). Cool.

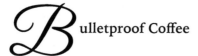 ulletproof Coffee

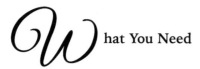 ervings: 1

Total Macro Nutrients:

- -0- g Net Carbs
- 1 g Total Protein
- 51 g Total Fats
- 463 Calories

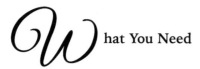 hat You Need

- MCT oil powder (2 tbsp.)
- Ghee or butter (2 tbsp.)
- Hot coffee (1.5 cups)

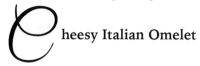

How To Prepare:

1. Prepare and pour the hot coffee into your blender.
2. Add in the powder and ghee/butter. Blend until frothy.
3. Serve in a large mug.

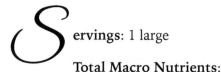

Cheesy Italian Omelet

Servings: 1 large

Total Macro Nutrients:

- 3 g Net Carbs
- 33 g Total Protein
- 36 g Total Fats
- 451 Calories

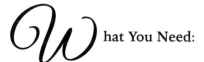

What You Need:

- Eggs (2)
- Water (1 tbsp.)
- Butter or ghee (1 tbsp.)
- Thin slices salami/prosciutto (3)
- Basil leaves (6)
- Mozzarella cheese slices (2 oz.)
- Thin slices of tomato (5)

- Pepper and salt (to taste)

*H*ow To Prepare:

1. Toss the ghee or butter in a frying pan using the medium heat setting to melt.
2. Whisk the water and eggs together. Pour into the hot pan and cook for about 30 seconds.
3. Spread out the meat slices over top of the egg followed by the cheese, tomatoes, and slices of basil. Season with the salt and pepper.
4. Cook approximately two minutes or until firm. Flip and cook an additional minute before folding in half.
5. Cover the pan and simmer over low heat.
6. When the center is done, add the omelet to a plate and serve.

Cream Cheese Eggs

*S*ervings: 1

Total Macro Nutrients:

- 3 g Net Carbs
- 15 g Total Protein
- 31 g Total Fats
- 341 Calories

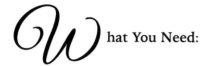

What You Need:

- Butter (1 tbsp.)
- Eggs (2)
- Soft cream cheese with chives (2 tbsp.)

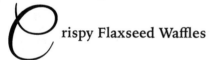

How to Prepare:

1. Preheat a skillet and melt the butter.
2. Whisk the eggs with the cream cheese.
3. Add to the pan and stir until done.

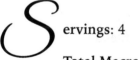

Crispy Flaxseed Waffles

Servings: 4

Total Macro Nutrients:

- 3 g Net Carbs
- 18.3 g Total Protein
- 42 g Total Fats
- 550 Calories

*W*hat You Need:

- Roughly ground flaxseed (2 cups)
- Baking powder - gluten-free (1 tbsp.)
- Sea salt (1 tsp.)
- Large eggs (5)
- Water (.5 cup)
- Avocado/Coconut/Extra-virgin olive oil (.33 cup)
- Ground cinnamon (2 tsp.)

*H*ow To Prepare:

1. Warm up the waffle maker on the countertop using the medium heat setting.
2. Combine the baking powder, sea salt, and flaxseeds in a mixing container. Whisk well and set aside.
3. In a blender, add the oil, water, and eggs. Blend for 30 seconds until foamy. Pour the mixture into the bowl with flaxseeds.
4. Stir until just incorporated and allow to rest for 3 minutes.
5. At that time, stir in the cinnamon and pour into the waffle maker.
6. Serve right away or place in the freezer for a couple of weeks.

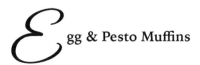

Egg & Pesto Muffins

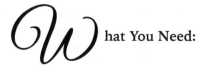

Servings: 10

Total Macro Nutrients:

- 1.2 g Net Carbs
- 6.9 g Total Protein
- 10.2 g Total Fats
- 125 Calories

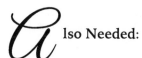

What You Need:

- Pesto (3 tbsp.)
- Frozen spinach (.66 cup)
- Pitted Kalamata olives (.5 cup)
- Chopped sun-dried tomatoes (.25 cup)
- Large eggs (6)
- Feta - soft goat cheese (4.4 oz.)
- Pepper & Himalayan salt (to your liking)

Also Needed:

- Muffin Tin
- Bowl cups

*H*ow To Prepare:

1. Set the oven temperature to 350° Fahrenheit.
2. Thaw and remove the excess liquid from the spinach (You can also blanch freshly picked spinach for one minute in boiling water. Transfer it to an ice bath to stop the cooking process.)
3. Chop the tomatoes and slice the olives.
4. Whisk in the pesto, salt, and pepper.
5. Divide the ingredients evenly into the cups - starting with the spinach, cheese, tomatoes, and olives. Blend in the pesto and egg mixture.
6. Bake 20 to 25 minutes or until browned.
7. When the muffins are done, place them on a cooling rack for a short time.
8. You can store the tasty breakfast treats in the fridge for five days or so.

Ham Muffins

*S*ervings: 12

Total Macro Nutrients:

- 1.5 g Net Carbs
- 10 g Total Protein
- 9 g Total Fats

- 129 Calories

What You Need:

- Ham (12 oz.)
- Green pepper (.25 cup)
- Celery (1 stalk)
- Pepper (1 tsp.)
- Onion powder (1 tsp.)
- Freshly chopped parsley (1 tbsp.)
- Minced chives (1 tbsp.)
- Dash of cayenne (1 dash)
- Shredded cheddar cheese (6 oz.)
- Eggs (3)

How To Prepare:

1. Line a rimmed baking sheet with foil. Spritz the muffin tins with cooking oil spray.
2. Mince the celery and green pepper. Finely mince the ham in a food processor. Combine all of the fixings.
3. Spoon into the muffin tins sitting on the baking tin.
4. Set the oven to 350° Fahrenheit. Bake for 30 to 35 minutes or until browned.

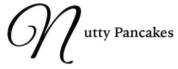

Nutty Pancakes

Servings: 2

Total Macro Nutrients:

- 9 g Net Carbs
- 27 g Total Protein
- 52 g Total Fats
- 625 Calories

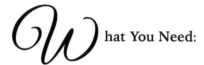

What You Need:

- Almond flour (10 tbsp.)
- Baking soda (.5 tsp.)
- Ground cinnamon (1 tsp.)
- Large eggs (3)
- Almond milk (.25 cup)
- Chopped nuts – ex. Hazelnuts (.25 cup)
- Unsweetened almond/preference nut butter (.25 cup)

How to Prepare:

1. Whisk all of the fixings in a container. Let the batter sit for 5-10 minutes for the flour will thicken.
2. Preheat a greased skillet (low-medium).
3. Measure out .25 cup portions of the batter in the frying pan.
4. Cook for 2-3 minutes per side.
5. Serve with the prepared almond butter drizzle.

 il-Free Blueberry Streusel Scones

 ervings: 12

Total Macro Nutrients:

- 3.3 g Net Carbs
- 0.6 g Total Protein
- 11.6 g Total Fats
- 145 Calories

 hat You Need For The Scones:

- Almond flour (2 cups)
- Baking powder (1 tsp.)
- Ground stevia leaf (.25 tsp.)
- Salt (1 pinch)
- Fresh blueberries (1 cup)
- Egg (1)
- Almond milk (2 tbsp.)

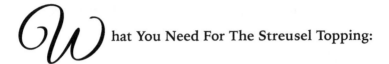

What You Need For The Streusel Topping:

- Egg white (1 tbsp.)
- Slivered almonds (.25 cup)
- Ground cinnamon (.5 tsp.)
- Stevia (1 pinch)

How To Prepare:

1. Warm up the oven to reach 375° Fahrenheit. Prepare a cookie sheet with parchment paper or use a silicone baking mat.
2. Combine all of the fixings for the streusel in a small mixing bowl.
3. In a large bowl, combine the flour, stevia, baking powder, and salt. Whisk well to mix.
4. Stir in the blueberries and cover with the flour mixture. Set to the side for now.
5. Whisk the egg and milk together and add with the flour mixture. Stir well. Knead the dough and shape into 12 small scones about ½-inch thick.
6. Place on the prepared pan and bake for 22 to 22 minutes.
7. Cool 10 minutes and serve.

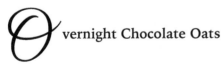

Overnight Chocolate Oats

. . .

*S*ervings: 4

Total Macro Nutrients:

- 3 g Net Carbs
- 4.9 g Total Protein
- 11.1 g Total Fats
- 139 Calories

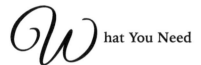 hat You Need

- Chopped walnuts (.33 cup)
- Chia seeds (.25 cup)
- MCT oil or powder (.25 cup) optional
- Cacao powder (2 tbsp.)
- Cacao nibs (2 tbsp.)
- Liquid stevia (4 drops) or Erythritol (2 tbsp.)
- Cinnamon (.5 tsp.)
- Finely ground sea salt (.25 tsp.)
- Non-dairy milk - your choice (2 cups)
- Vanilla extract (1 tsp.)

*H*ow To Prepare:

1. Add the MCT oil, chia seeds, walnuts, cacao nibs, cacao

powder, ground cinnamon, sweetener of choice, and sea salt. Place in an airtight container large enough to hold at least four cups.

2. Rotate the ingredients in the container until fully coated.
3. Pour in the milk and add the vanilla extract. Stir until well-mixed.
4. Securely place a cover on the jar and refrigerate for at least 12 hours.
5. When time to eat, stir well and divide between four bowls to serve.

 aspberry Breakfast Pudding Bowl

 ervings: 3 (.5 cup each)

Total Macro Nutrients:

- 5.7 g Net Carbs
- 3.2 g Total Protein
- 34.2 g Total Fats
- 328 Calories

 hat You Need:

- Full-fat coconut milk (1.5 cups)
- Frozen raspberries (1 cup)
- MCT oil (.25 cup)
- Chia seeds (2 tbsp.)

- Apple cider vinegar (1 tbsp.)
- Alcohol-free stevia (3 drops)
- Vanilla extract (1 tsp.)
- Optional: Collagen (1 scoop)

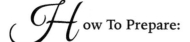 ow To Prepare:

1. Combine all of the pudding fixings in the bowl of the food processor or jug of the blender.
2. Combine until creamy smooth.
3. Serve in a bowl (¾-cup size) and top with your favorites.
4. Serve with almonds, shredded coconut, fresh berries or hemp hearts. Remember to add additional carbs.

 ausage - Eggs & Broccoli with Cheese

 ervings: 6

Total Macro Nutrients:

- 4.21 g Net Carbs
- 26.1 g Total Protein
- 38.9 g Total Fats
- 484 Calories

*W*hat You Need

- Medium head of broccoli (1)
- Low-carb sausage links (12. oz. pkg.)
- Shredded cheddar cheese (1 cup - divided)
- Eggs (10)
- Whipping cream (.75 cup)
- Minced garlic cloves (2)
- Pepper (.25 tsp.)
- Salt (.5 tsp.)
- Suggested Size: 6-quart slow cooker

*H*ow To Prepare:

1. Chop the broccoli. Mince the garlic and slice the sausage. Grease the pot with some non-stick cooking spray.
2. Layer the broccoli, sausage, and cheese in two-layer segments (6 layers total).
3. Combine the whipping cream, whisked eggs, salt, pepper, and garlic until well mixed. Add to the layered fixings.
4. Secure the lid and cook for two to three hours on high or for four to five hours on the low setting. The edges are browned, and the center is set when it is ready to serve.
5. Note: Make your own creation but count the carbs.

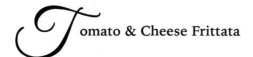

Tomato & Cheese Frittata

Servings: 2

Total Macro Nutrients:

- 6 g Net Carbs
- 27 g Total Protein
- 33 g Total Fats
- 435 Calories

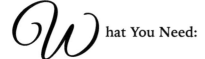

What You Need:

- Eggs (6)
- Soft cheese (3.5 oz. - .66 cup)
- White onion (.5 of 1 medium)
- Halved cherry tomatoes (.66 cup)
- Chopped herbs - ex. Chives or basil (2 tbsp.)
- Ghee or butter (1 tbsp.)
- Optional Garnish: Feta

How to Prepare:

1. Warm up the oven broiler temperature to 400° Fahrenheit.
2. Arrange the onions on a greased - hot iron skillet. Cook with either the ghee or butter until lightly browned.
3. In another dish, whisk the eggs with the salt, pepper, or add some herbs of your choice. Add to the pan of onions, cooking until the edges get crispy.
4. Top with the cheese if you choose, and a few diced tomatoes. Put the pan in the broiler for five to seven minutes or until done.
5. Enjoy piping hot or let cool down.
6. Note: You can purge all of your leftover veggies into the recipe.
7. Divide into two equal portions. Serve either hot or cold.

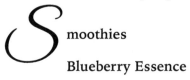 moothies

Blueberry Essence

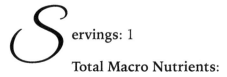 ervings: 1

Total Macro Nutrients:

- 3 g Net Carbs
- 31 g Total Protein
- 21 g Total Fats
- 343 Calories

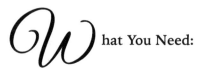 hat You Need:

- Coconut milk (1 cup)
- Blueberries (.25 cup)
- Vanilla Essence (1 tsp.)
- MCT oil (1 tsp.)
- Ice cubes (2-3)

How To Prepare:

1. For a quick burst of energy, combine each of the fixings in a blender.
2. Puree until it reaches the desired consistency.
3. Pour and serve into a chilled glass.

Mocha 5-Minute Smoothie

Servings: 3

Total Macro Nutrients:

- 4 g Net Carbs
- 3 g Total Protein
- 16 g Total Fats
- 176 Calories

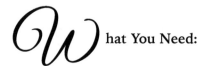# What You Need:

- Avocado (1)
- Coconut milk – from the can (.5 cup)
- Unsweetened almond milk (1.5 cups)
- Instant coffee crystals – regular or decaffeinated (2 tsp.)
- Vanilla extract (1 tsp.)
- Erythritol blend/granulated stevia (3 tbsp.)
- Unsweetened cocoa powder (3 tbsp.)

How To Prepare:

1. Slice the avocado in half. Discard the pit and remove most of the center. Add it along with the rest of the fixings into a blender.
2. Mix until it's like you like it. Serve in three chilled glasses.

LUNCHEON SPECIALTIES

- *Bacon & Shrimp Risotto*
- *Bacon Burger Cabbage Stir Fry*
- *Baked Zucchini Noodles With Feta*
- Cabbage Rolls - Slow Cooker
- *Cheesy Bacon-Wrapped Hot Dogs*
- *Chicken Nuggets*
- *Coleslaw Stuffed Wraps*
- *Creamy Basil Baked Sausage*
- *Creamy Salmon & Pasta*
- *Ground Beef Pizza*
- *Omelet Wrap With Avocado & Salmon*
- *Quick & Easy Taco Casserole*
- *Shrimp Alfredo*
- *Spicy Mexican Lettuce Wraps*
- *Spinach & Ham Mini Quiche*

SOUP CHOICES

- *Asiago Tomato Soup*
- *Broccoli & Cheese Soup*
- *Creamy Chicken & Garlic Soup*
- *No-Beans Chili*

LUNCHEON SPECIALTIES

Bacon & Shrimp Risotto

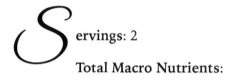

ervings: 2

Total Macro Nutrients:

- 5.3 g Net Carbs
- 23.7 g Total Protein
- 9.4 g Total Fats
- 224 Calories

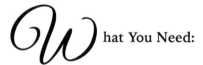

hat You Need:

- Chopped bacon (4 slices)
- Daikon - winter radish (2 cups)
- Dry white wine (2 tbsp.)
- Chicken stock (.25 cup)
- Minced garlic (1 clove)
- Ground pepper (as desired)
- Chopped parsley (2 tbsp.)

- Cooked shrimp (4 oz.)

$\mathcal{H}$ow To Prepare:

1. Peel and slice the radish, mince the garlic, and chop the bacon. Remove as much water as possible from the daikon once it's shredded.
2. On the stovetop, heat up a saucepan using the medium heat temperature setting. Toss in the bacon and fry until it's crispy. Leave the drippings in the pan and remove the bacon with a slotted spoon to drain.
3. Add the stock, wine, daikon, salt, pepper, and garlic into the pan. Simmer for 6-8 minutes until most of the liquid is absorbed.
4. Fold in the bacon (saving a few bits for the topping), and shrimp along with the parsley. Serve.
5. *Tip*: If you cannot find the daikon, just substitute it using shredded cauliflower.

$\mathcal{B}$acon Burger Cabbage Stir Fry

$\mathcal{S}$ervings: 10

Total Macro Nutrients:

- 4.5 g Net Carbs
- 31.9 g Total Protein
- 22 g Total Fats

- 357 Calories

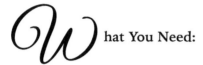

What You Need:

- Ground beef (1 lb.)
- Bacon (1 lb.)
- Small onion (1)
- Minced cloves of garlic (3)
- Cabbage (1 lb. - 1 small head)
- Black pepper (.25 tsp.)
- Sea salt (.5 tsp.)

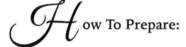

How To Prepare:

1. Dice the bacon and onion.
2. Combine the beef and bacon in a wok or large skillet. Prepare until done and store in a bowl to keep warm.
3. Mince the garlic and toss with the onion into the hot grease. Add the cabbage and stir-fry until wilted. Blend in the meat and combine. Sprinkle with the pepper and salt as desired.

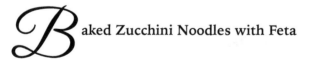

Baked Zucchini Noodles with Feta

. . .

*S*ervings: 3

Total Macro Nutrients:

- 5 g Net Carbs
- 4 g Total Protein
- 8 g Total Fats
- 105 Calories

*W*hat You Need:

- Quartered plum tomato (1)
- Spiralized zucchini (2)
- Feta cheese (8 cubes)
- Pepper and salt (1 tsp. each)
- Olive oil (1 tbsp.)

*H*ow To Prepare:

1. Lightly grease a roasting pan with a spritz of oil.
2. Set the oven temperature to reach 375° Fahrenheit.
3. Slice the noodles with a spiralizer and add to the prepared pan along with the olive oil and tomatoes. Sprinkle with the pepper and salt.
4. Bake for 10 to 15 minutes. Transfer from the oven and add the cheese cubes, tossing to combine. Serve.

Cabbage Rolls - Slow Cooker

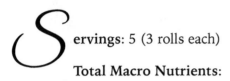

ervings: 5 (3 rolls each)

Total Macro Nutrients:

- 4.2 g Net Carbs
- 35 g Total Protein
- 25 g Total Fats
- 481 Calories

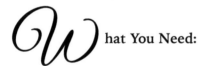

hat You Need:

- Corned beef (3.5 lb.)
- Large savoy cabbage leaves (15)
- White wine (.25 cup)
- Coffee (.25 cup)
- Large lemon (1)
- Medium sliced onion (1)
- Rendered bacon fat (1 tbsp.)
- Erythritol (1 tbsp.)
- Yellow mustard (1 tbsp.)
- Large bay leaf (1)
- Kosher salt (2 tsp.)
- Worcestershire sauce (2 tsp.)
- Cloves (.25 tsp.)
- Allspice (.25 tsp.)
- Whole peppercorns (1 tsp.)
- Mustard seeds (1 tsp.)

- Red pepper flakes (.5 tsp.)

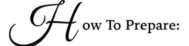

How To Prepare:

1. Pour the liquids, corned beef, and spices into the cooker. Set the timer for six hours using the low setting.
2. Prepare a pot of boiling water. When the timer on the slow cooker buzzes, add the leaves along with the sliced onion to the water for two to three minutes. Transfer the leaves to a cold-water bath. Blanch them for three to four minutes. Continue boiling the onion.
3. Use a paper towel to dry the leaves. Add the onions and beef.
4. Roll up the cabbage leaves. Drizzle with freshly squeezed lemon juice. Serve any time.

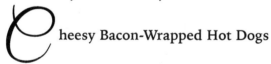

Cheesy Bacon-Wrapped Hot Dogs

Servings: 6

Total Macro Nutrients:

- 2.1 g Net Carbs
- 13.6 g Total Protein
- 19.3 g Total Fats
- 283 Calories

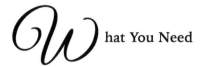 What You Need

- Bacon slices (12)
- Large beef hot dogs (6)
- Onion (.5 tsp.)
- Garlic (.5 tsp.)
- Pepper & salt (to your liking)
- Cheddar cheese (2 oz.)

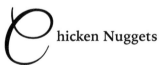 ow To Prepare:

1. Warm up the oven temperature to reach 400° Fahrenheit.
2. Slice each of the hot dogs (not all the way through) and insert the cheese. Wrap the hot dogs with two bacon slices each and secure with a toothpick.
3. Add the seasoning to a dish and roll the dogs through it.
4. Bake 35-40 minutes. Serve with your favorite side dishes or as a snack.
5. Note: You can adjust the time and cook them as using small chunks for variation

Chicken Nuggets

· · ·

*S*ervings: 6

Total Macro Nutrients:

- 2 g Net Carbs
- 18 g Total Protein
- 17 g Total Fats
- 243 Calories

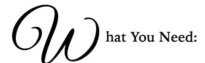 hat You Need:

- Cooked chicken (2 cups)
- Cream cheese (8 oz.)
- Egg (1)
- Garlic salt (1 tsp.)
- Almond flour (.25 cup)

*H*ow To Prepare:

1. Set the oven temperature to 350° Fahrenheit.
2. Lightly grease a baking pan with a spritz of cooking oil spray. You can also use a layer of parchment paper.
3. Shred the chicken using a food processor or by hand. (Try using a combination of dark and light meat.)
4. Combine the rest of the fixings and mix well.
5. Scoop the nugget mixture onto the prepared baking tin.
6. Bake until firm and slightly browned (12-14 min.).

Coleslaw Stuffed Wraps

 ervings: 4 - Total of 16 wraps

Total Macro Nutrients:

- 3.1 g Net Carbs
- 33 g Total Protein
- 50 g Total Fats
- 609 Calories

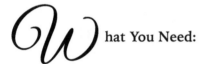 hat You Need:

- Green onions (.5 cup)
- Red cabbage (3 cups)
- Keto-friendly mayonnaise (.75 cup)
- Apple cider vinegar (2 tsp.)
- Sea salt (.25 tsp.)

 hat You Need for the Wraps and Other Fillings:

- Ground beef/turkey/pork/chicken– cooked & chilled (1 lb.)
- Collard leaves (16)
- Packed alfalfa sprouts (.33 cup)
- Toothpicks

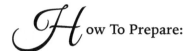

How To Prepare:

1. Prepare the meat of choice in a frying pan. Thinly slice the cabbage. Remove the stems from the collards and dice the onions. Add all of the fixings in a large mixing container and stir well.
2. Add a spoonful of the coleslaw on the far edge of the first collard leaf (the side that hasn't been cut). Add the meat and the sprouts.
3. Roll and tuck the sides and insert toothpicks at an angle to hold them together. Continue until all are done. Serve.

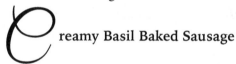

Creamy Basil Baked Sausage

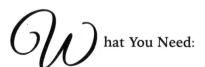

Servings: 12

Total Macro Nutrients:

- 4 g Net Carbs
- 23 g Total Protein
- 23 g Total Fats
- 316 Calories

What You Need:

- Italian sausage - pork/turkey or chicken (3 lb.)
- Cream cheese (8 oz.)
- Heavy cream (.25 cup)
- Basil pesto (.25 cup)
- Mozzarella (8 oz.)

How To Prepare:

1. Warm up the oven to reach 400° Fahrenheit. Lightly spritz a casserole dish with cooking oil spray. Add the sausage to the dish and bake for 30 minutes.
2. Combine the heavy cream, pesto, and cream cheese.
3. Once the sauce is done, spread the sauce over the casserole and top it off with the cheese.
4. Bake for another 10 minutes. The sausage should reach 160° Fahrenheit in the center when checked with a meat thermometer.
5. You can also broil for 3 minutes to brown the cheesy layer.

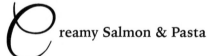

Creamy Salmon & Pasta

Servings: 2

Total Macro Nutrients:

- 3 g Net Carbs
- 21 g Total Protein
- 42 g Total Fats

- 470 Calories

What You Need:

- Zucchini (2)
- Coconut oil (2 tbsp.)
- Smoked salmon (8 oz.)
- Keto-friendly mayonnaise (.25 cup)

How to Prepare:

1. Use a peeler or spiralizer to make noodle-like strands from the zucchini.
2. Warm up the oil over the medium-high temperature setting.
3. When hot, add the salmon and sauté 2-3 minutes until golden brown.
4. Stir in the noodles and sauté 1-2 more minutes.
5. When it's time to eat, just stir in the mayo and divide the pasta between two dishes.

Ground Beef Pizza

. . .

*S*ervings: 4

Total Macro Nutrients:

- 2 g Net Carbs
- 44 g Total Protein
- 45 g Total Fats
- 610 Calories

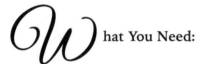

hat You Need:

- Large eggs (2)
- Ground beef (20 oz.)
- Pepperoni slices (28)
- Shredded cheddar cheese (.5 cup)
- Pizza sauce (.5 cup)
- Mozzarella cheese (4 oz.)
- Also Needed: 1 Cast iron skillet

*H*ow To Prepare:

1. Fold in the eggs, beef, and seasonings. Place in the skillet to form the crust for the pizza. Bake about 15 minutes or until the meat is done.
2. Take it out and add the sauce, cheese, and toppings.

3. Place the pizza back in the oven a few minutes until the cheese has melted.

 melet Wrap with Avocado & Salmon

 ervings: 2

Total Macro Nutrients:

- 5.8 g Net Carbs
- 37 g Total Protein
- 67 g Total Fats
- 765 Calories

 hat You Need:

- Large eggs (3)
- Smoked salmon (1.8 oz.)
- Average-sized avocado (3.5 oz. or .5 of 1)
- Spring onion (1)
- Cream cheese - full-fat (2 tbsp.)
- Freshly chopped chives (2 tbsp.)
- Butter or ghee (1 tbsp.)

How To Prepare:

1. In a mixing bowl, add a pinch of pepper and salt along with the eggs. Whisk well. Fold in the chives and cream cheese.
2. Prepare the salmon and avocado, peel and slice.

3. In a skillet, add the butter or ghee to melt. Add the egg mixture and cook until fluffy. Put the omelet on a serving dish and spoon the combination of cheese over it.

4. Sprinkle the onion, prepared avocado, and salmon into the wrap.

5. Close the prepared wrap and serve.

Quick & Easy Taco Casserole

Servings: 6

Total Macro Nutrients:

- 6 g Net Carbs
- 45 g Total Protein
- 18 g Total Fats
- 367 Calories

What You Need:

- Ground Turkey or Beef (1.5-2 lb.)
- Taco seasoning (2 tbsp.)
- Shredded cheddar cheese (8 oz.)
- Cottage cheese (16 oz.)
- Salsa (1 cup)

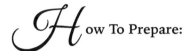

How To Prepare:

1. Warm up the oven to reach 400° Fahrenheit.
2. Combine the taco seasoning and ground meat in a casserole dish. Bake for 20 minutes.
3. Combine the salsa and both kinds of cheese. Set aside for now.
4. Carefully remove the casserole dish from the oven and drain away the cooking juices from the meat.
5. Break the meat into small pieces and mash with a potato masher or fork.
6. Sprinkle with the cheese and place in the oven for 15-20 more minutes until the top is browned.

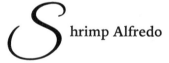

Shrimp Alfredo

Servings: 4

Total Macro Nutrients:

- 6.5 g Net Carbs
- 22.9 g Total Protein
- 17.6 g Total Fats
- 298 Calories

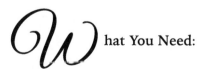

What You Need:

- Raw shrimp (1 lb.)
- Salted butter (1 tbsp.)
- Cubed cream cheese (4 oz.)
- Whole milk (.5 cup)
- Salt (1 tsp.)
- Dried basil (1 tsp.)
- Garlic powder (1 tbsp.)
- Shredded parmesan cheese (.5 cup)
- Baby kale or spinach (.25 cup)
- Whole sun-dried tomatoes (5 cut in strips)

How To Prepare:

1. Heat up the butter using the medium heat setting in a skillet.
2. Toss in the shrimp and lower the heat to medium-low. After 30 seconds, flip the shrimp and cook until slightly pink. Blend in the cream cheese.
3. Increase the heat and pour in the milk. Stir frequently.
4. Sprinkle with the salt, basil, and garlic. Empty the parmesan cheese in and mix well.
5. Simmer until the sauce has thickened. Lastly, fold in the kale/spinach and dried tomatoes. Serve steaming hot.

Spicy Mexican Lettuce Wraps

. . .

*S*ervings: 4

Total Macro Nutrients:

- 5.4 g Net Carbs
- 15 g Total Protein
- 16 g Total Fats
- 233 Calories

*W*hat You Need:

- Chicken breasts (2)
- Red pepper (1)
- Hot or mild chili powder (.25 tsp. or as desired)
- Avocado (1)
- Olive oil (2 tbsp.)
- Cheddar cheese (.25 cup)
- Large lettuce leaves (4)
- Medium white onion (1)
- Keto-friendly sour cream - to garnish (1 tbsp.)

*H*ow To Prepare:

1. Dice the pepper, onion, and chicken.
2. Warm up the oil in a skillet on the stovetop. Cook the chicken using the high setting. Stir in the onion, chili powder, and pepper. Simmer 10 to 15 minutes.
3. Slice the avocado and grate the cheese. Portion the mixture

into each of the leaves and add a spoon of sour cream. Sprinkle with the pepper and refrigerate until ready to eat.

Spinach & Ham Mini Quiche

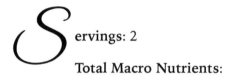

ervings: 2

Total Macro Nutrients:

- 2 g Net Carbs
- 20 g Total Protein
- 13 g Total Fats
- 210 Calories

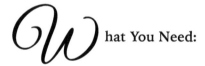

hat You Need:

- Diced ham (4) slices
- Whisked eggs (3)
- Chopped spinach (.75 cup)
- Chopped leek (.25 cup)
- Coconut milk (.25 cup)
- Baking powder (.5 tsp.)
- Pepper & salt (to your liking)

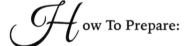

ow To Prepare:

1. Warm up the oven temperature to 350° Fahrenheit.

2. Combine all of the fixings in a large mixing container.
3. Pour the mixture into tart pans or four small mini quiche pans.
4. Bake 15 minutes. Serve.

 Soup Choices

Asiago Tomato Soup

 Servings: 4

Total Macro Nutrients:

- 8.75 g Net Carbs
- 9.3 g Total Protein
- 25.8 g Total Fats
- 301.5 Calories

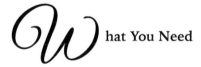 **W**hat You Need

- Tomato paste (1 small can)
- Minced garlic (1 tsp.)
- Oregano (1 tsp.)
- Heavy whipping cream (1 cup)
- Water (.25 cup)
- Pepper and salt (as desired)
- Asiago cheese (.75 cup)

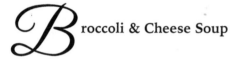# How To Prepare:

1. Pour the minced garlic and tomato paste in a Dutch oven and add the cream. Gently whisk.
2. As it begins to boil, blend in small amounts of cheese. Pour in the water and simmer 4-5 minutes.
3. Serve with pepper as desired.

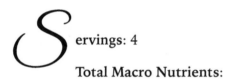# Broccoli & Cheese Soup

Servings: 4

Total Macro Nutrients:

- 9.88 g Net Carbs
- 23.9 g Total Protein
- 52.3 g Total Fats
- 561 Calories

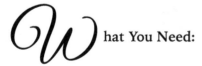# What You Need:

- Small diced onion (1)
- Chopped broccoli (4 cups)
- Vegetable stock (1.5 cups)
- Minced garlic (1 tsp.)

- Shredded sharp cheddar cheese (3 cups)
- Pepper & salt (to your liking)
- Heavy cream (.75 cup)

*H*ow To Prepare:

1. Use the medium heat setting on the stovetop to warm a skillet. Toss in the broccoli, onions, and garlic. Sauté for about five minutes.
2. Once boiling, cover, and simmer for another ten minutes.
3. Pour in the heavy cream and cook for three to five minutes.
4. Fold in the cheese and stir until creamy smooth or around one to two minutes. Give it a shake of salt and pepper. Serve.

Creamy Chicken & Garlic Soup

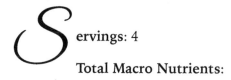 ervings: 4

Total Macro Nutrients:

- 2 g Net Carbs
- 18 g Total Protein
- 25 g Total Fats
- 307 Calories

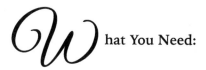 hat You Need:

- Butter (2 tbsp.)
- Chicken (1 large breast or 2 cups shredded)
- Cubed cream cheese (4 oz.)
- Garlic seasoning (2 tbsp.)
- Chicken broth (14.5 oz.)
- Salt (to your liking)
- Heavy cream (.25 cup)

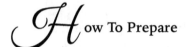ow To Prepare

1. Heat up a saucepan and melt the butter using the medium heat setting.
2. Shred and add the chicken. Toss and fold in the cream cheese and seasoning.
3. When melted, add the heavy cream and broth.
4. Lower the heat setting once the cheese and broth start boiling. Simmer for 3-4 minutes. Season as desired.

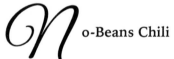o-Beans Chili

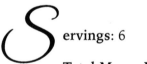ervings: 6

Total Macro Nutrients:

- 5 g Net Carbs
- 26 g Total Protein
- 14 g Total Fats
- 263 Calories

*W*hat You Need:

- Water (3 cups)
- Ground beef 1.5 lb.)
- Cumin (.75 tsp.)
- Black pepper (.75 tsp.)
- Cinnamon (.25 tsp.)
- Minced garlic cloves (2)
- Chopped onion (.25 cup)
- Worcestershire sauce (1 tsp.)
- Bay leaves (3)
- Chili powder (2 tbsp.)
- Salt (1.5 tsp.)
- Allspice (.5 tsp.)
- Red pepper (.5 tsp.)
- Tomato paste (6 oz.)
- Sliced black olives (2.25 oz.)
- Finely chopped chili peppers (.25 cup)

*H*ow To Prepare:

1. Break apart the ground beef in a large stew pot on the stovetop. Drain away the juices.
2. Combine with the rest of the fixings. Bring to a boil.
3. Simmer two hours and serve.

DINNER FAVORITES

POULTRY OPTIONS

Chicken with Yogurt & Mango Sauce

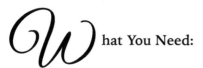

Servings: 4

Total Macro Nutrients:

- 3 g Net Carbs
- 54 g Total Protein
- 6 g Total Fats
- 296 Calories

What You Need:

- Chicken breasts (4)
- Plain yogurt (.25 cup)
- Mango (.25 cup)
- Small red onion (1)
- Ground ginger (1 tsp.)
- Freshly cracked black pepper and salt (to your liking)

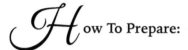 ow To Prepare:

1. Warm up the oven to 350° Fahrenheit.
2. Dice the chicken, mango, and onion.
3. Fry the chicken in the oil until browned. Toss in the mango and onion. Cook for another three minutes.
4. Stir in the yogurt. Dust with the salt and pepper.
5. Add to a baking dish and bake for 25 to 30 minutes.
6. Serve when ready.

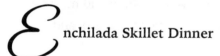 nchilada Skillet Dinner

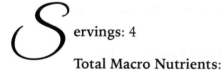 ervings: 4

Total Macro Nutrients:

- 7 g Net Carbs
- 36 g Total Protein
- 30 g Total Fats
- 455 Calories

𝒲hat You Need:

- Small yellow onion (1)
- Ground beef (1.5 lb.)
- Red enchilada sauce (.66 cup)
- Chopped green onions (8)
- Diced Roma tomatoes (2)
- Shredded cheddar cheese (4 oz.)
- Optional: Freshly chopped cilantro (to taste)

ℋow To Prepare:

1. Use a wok or skillet to sauté the yellow onion and meat. Drain the juices and add the green onions, tomato, and enchilada sauce.
2. Once it starts to boil, simmer for about 5 minutes. Sprinkle with the salt and cheese. Continue cooking until the cheese has melted.
3. Stir in the cilantro. Serve over chopped lettuce and serving of sour cream. Add the extra carbs and enjoy.

ℋerbal Green Beans & Chicken

. . .

*S*ervings: 3

Total Macro Nutrients:

- 4 g Net Carbs
- 19 g Total Protein
- 11 g Total Fats
- 196 Calories

*W*hat You Need:

- Olive oil (2 tbsp.)
- Trimmed green beans (1 cup)
- Whole chicken breasts (2)
- Halved cherry tomatoes (8)
- Italian seasoning (1 tbsp.)
- Salt and pepper (1 tsp.)

*H*ow To Prepare:

1. Warm up a skillet using the medium heat temperature setting. Pour in the oil.
2. Sprinkle the chicken with the pepper, salt, and Italian seasoning.
3. Arrange in the skillet and cook for 10 minutes per side or until well done.

4. Add the tomatoes and beans. Simmer another 5 to 7 minutes and serve.

Lemon Parsley Buttered Chicken

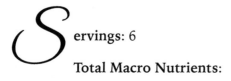

ervings: 6

Total Macro Nutrients:

- 1 g Net Carbs
- 29 g Total Protein
- 18 g Total Fats
- 300 Calories

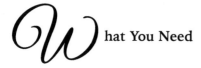

hat You Need

- Whole roasting chicken (5-6 lb.)
- Black pepper (.25 tsp.)
- Kosher salt (.5 tsp.)
- Water (1 cup)
- Thinly sliced lemon (1)
- Ghee/butter (4 tbsp.)
- Chopped fresh parsley (2 tbsp.)
- Also Needed: Slow cooker

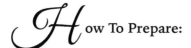

ow To Prepare:

1. Remove the innards (discard) and rinse the chicken. Dry it off with some paper towels and rub it with the pepper and salt.
2. Arrange the whole chicken in the slow cooker and pour the water into the pot. Set the cooker for 3 hours or when the bird reaches an internal temperature of 165° Fahrenheit at the thickest segment of the thigh.
3. Add the lemon slices, butter, and parsley into the cooker for about ten minutes.
4. To Serve: Pour the parsley butter over the chicken and enjoy. Garnish with other toppings of your choosing.

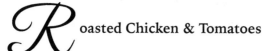

oasted Chicken & Tomatoes

ervings: 2

Total Macro Nutrients:

- 5 g Net Carbs
- 16 g Total Protein
- 16 g Total Fats
- 233 Calories

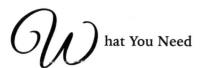

hat You Need

- Plum tomatoes (2 quartered)
- Chicken legs – bone-in with skin (2)
- Paprika (1 tsp.)
- Ground oregano (1 tsp.)
- Balsamic vinegar (1 tbsp.)
- Olive oil (1 tbsp.)

*H*ow To Prepare:

1. Set the oven temperature setting to 350° Fahrenheit. Grease a roasting pan with a spritz of oil.
2. Rinse and lightly dab the chicken legs dry with a paper towel. Prepare using the oil and vinegar over the skin. Season with the paprika and oregano.
3. Arrange the legs in the pan along with the tomatoes around the edges.
4. Cover with a layer of foil and bake one hour. Baste to prevent the chicken from drying out.
5. Discard the foil and increase the temperature to 425° Fahrenheit. Bake 15 to 30 minutes more until browned and the juices run clear.
6. Serve with a side salad.

Smothered Chicken in Creamy Onion Sauce

*S*ervings: 4

Total Macro Nutrients (No Veggies):

- 3.3 g Net Carbs

- 38.4 g Total Protein
- 26 g Total Fats
- 400 Calories

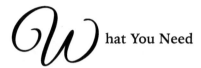hat You Need

- Whole green spring onion (1)
- Butter (2 tbsp. or 1-oz.)
- Chicken breast halves (4)
- Sour cream (8 oz.)
- Sea salt (.5 tsp.)

How To Prepare:

1. Remove all skin and bones from the chicken breasts.
2. Warm up a skillet using the med-high setting to melt the butter.
3. Reduce the setting to med-low and arrange the chicken in the skillet with the butter. Place a lid on the pan and cook about ten minutes.
4. Chop the onion using the white and green sections. Flip the chicken breasts. Cover and simmer another eight or nine minutes or until done.
5. Combine the onion and cook an additional one or two minutes.
6. Take it off the burner. Blend in the sour cream and salt.

7. Wait for about five minutes. Mix well with your favorite veggies and serve.

 tuffed Chicken with Bacon & Asparagus

 ervings: 4

Total Macro Nutrients:

- 2 g Net Carbs
- 32 g Total Protein
- 25 g Total Fats
- 377 Calories

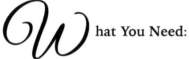 **hat You Need:**

- Bacon pieces (.5 lb. or 8 slices)
- Chicken tenders (8 or about 1 lb.)
- Salt (.5 tsp.)
- Black pepper (.25 tsp.)
- Asparagus spears (12 or about .5 lb.)

𝓗 **ow To Prepare:**

1. Warm up the oven to reach 400° Fahrenheit.
2. Prepare a baking sheet and lay out two slices of bacon. Place the chicken tenders on top of that and sprinkle with a dusting of salt and pepper.
3. Add three spears of the asparagus and wrap with the bacon and chicken to hold it all together. Continue the process and bake for 40 minutes. The bacon should be crispy and the asparagus tender.

 ther Choices

Bacon Cheeseburger

 ervings: 12

Total Macro Nutrients:

- 0.8 g Net Carbs
- 27 g Total Protein
- 41 g Total Fats
- 489 Calories

 hat You Need

- Low-sodium bacon (16 oz. pkg.)
- Ground beef (3 lb.)
- Eggs (2)
- Medium chopped onion (.5 of 1)
- Shredded cheddar cheese (8 oz.)

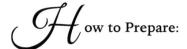

How to Prepare:

1. Fry the bacon and chop to bits. Shred the cheese and dice the onion.
2. Combine the mixture with the beef and blend in the whisked eggs.
3. Prepare 24 burgers and grill them the way you like them. You can make a double-decker since they are small. If you like a larger burger, you can just make 12 burgers as a single-decker.

Baked Marinara Spaghetti Squash

Servings: 4

Total Macro Nutrients:

- 5 g Net Carbs
- 3 g Total Protein
- 6 g Total Fats
- 92 Calories

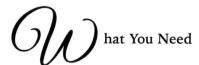

What You Need

- Marinara sauce – no sugar (.5 cup)

- Spaghetti squash (1)
- Sliced mushrooms (.5 cup)
- Salt and black pepper (1 tsp. each)
- Olive oil (1 tbsp.)
- Shredded mozzarella cheese (.25 cup)

 ow To Prepare:

1. Program the oven setting to 375 °Fahrenheit.
2. Cut the squash in half and discard the seeds.
3. Drizzle with the oil and sprinkle with the pepper and salt.
4. Flip onto the baking sheet (cut side down).
5. Bake 35 minutes until the squash is removed with a fork easily. If it's not done, cook another 10 minutes.
6. Serve.

 elicious Short Ribs

ervings: 4

Total Macro Nutrients:

- 2.5 g Net Carbs
- 25.7 g Total Protein
- 62 g Total Fats
- 685 Calories

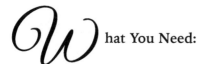

What You Need:

- Rice vinegar (2 tbsp.)
- Fish sauce (2 tbsp.)
- Keto-friendly soy sauce (.25 cup)
- Beef short ribs (6 - 4 oz. each)
- Red pepper flakes (.5 tsp.)
- Sesame seeds (.5 tsp.)
- Onion powder (.5 tsp.)
- Minced garlic (.5 tsp.)
- Ground ginger (1 tsp.)
- Salt (1 tbsp.)
- Cardamom (.25 tsp.)

How to Prepare:

1. Mix the fish sauce, vinegar, and alternative soy sauce.
2. Arrange the ribs in a dish with high sides. Add the sauce and marinate for up to one hour.
3. Combine all of the spices together. Take the ribs from the dish and sprinkle with the rub.
4. Warm up the grill (medium-high) and cook for 3 to 5 minutes on each side. Put the ribs in a platter and serve.

 ## Garlic & Thyme Lamb Chops

. . .

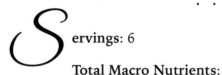

ervings: 6

Total Macro Nutrients:

- 1 g Net Carbs
- 14 g Total Protein
- 21 g Total Fats
- 252 Calories

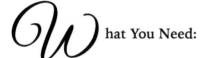

hat You Need:

- Lamb chops (6 - 4 oz.)
- Whole garlic cloves (4)
- Thyme sprigs (2)
- Ground thyme (1 tsp.)
- Olive oil (3 tbsp.)
- Black Pepper and Salt (1 tsp. each)

ow To Prepare:

1. Warm up a skillet using the medium heat setting. Once it's hot, add the olive oil.
2. Season the chops with the spices (pepper, thyme, and salt).
3. Arrange the chops in the skillet along with the garlic and sprigs of thyme.
4. Sauté about 3-4 minutes on each side and serve.

Ginger Sesame Salmon

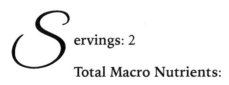

ervings: 2

Total Macro Nutrients:

- 2.5 g Net Carbs
- 33 g Total Protein
- 23.5 g Total Fats
- 370 Calories

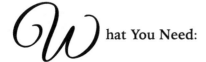

hat You Need:

- Salmon fillet (10 oz.)
- Sesame oil (2 tsp.)
- White wine (2 tbsp.)
- Soy sauce (2 tbsp.)
- Minced ginger (1-2 tsp.)
- Rice vinegar (1 tbsp.)
- Sugar-free ketchup (1 tbsp.)
- Fish sauce - ex. Red Boat (1 tbsp.)

ow To Prepare:

1. Combine all of the fixings in a plastic container with a tight-fitting lid, omitting the ketchup, oil, and wine for now. Marinade for about 10-15 minutes.

2. On the stovetop, prepare a skillet using the high heat temperature setting and pour in the oil. Add the fish when it's hot with the skin side facing down.
3. Brown both sides for three to four minutes. When you flip it over, pour in the marinated juices and simmer. Arrange the fish on two dinner plates.
4. Add the wine and ketchup to the pan and simmer five minutes until it's reduced. Serve with your favorite side dish.

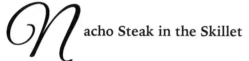 acho Steak in the Skillet

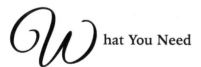 ervings: 5

Total Macro Nutrients:

- 6 g Net Carbs
- 19 g Total Protein
- 31 g Total Fats
- 385 Calories

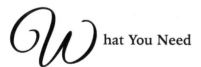 hat You Need

- Cauliflower (1.5 lb.)
- Turmeric (.5 turmeric)
- Chili powder (1 tsp.)
- Butter (1 tbsp.)
- Beef round tip steak (8 oz.)

- Melted refined coconut oil (.33 cup)
- Shredded cheddar cheese (1 oz.)
- Shredded Monterey Jack cheese (1 oz.)

Optional Garnishes:

- Sour cream (.33 cup)
- Canned - jalapeno slices (1 oz.)
- Avocado (approx. 5 oz.)

How To Prepare:

1. Warm up the oven temperature to 400° Fahrenheit.
2. Prepare the cauliflower into chip-like shapes.
3. Combine the turmeric, chili powder, and coconut oil in a mixing dish.
4. Toss in the cauliflower and add it to a baking tin. Set the baking timer for 20 to 25 minutes.
5. Over med-high heat in a cast iron skillet, add the butter. Cook until both sides of the meat is done, flipping just once. Let it rest for 5-10 minutes. Thinly slice and sprinkle with some pepper and salt.
6. When done, transfer the florets to the skillet and add the steak strips. Top it off with the cheese and bake for 5-10 more minutes.
7. Serve with your favorite garnish.
8. Count the carbs for the added garnishes.

Pan Fried Cod

. . .

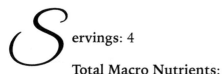

ervings: 4

Total Macro Nutrients:

- 1 g Net Carbs
- 21 g Total Protein
- 7 g Total Fats
- 160 Calories

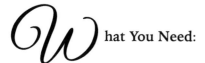

hat You Need:

- Ghee (3 tbsp.)
- Cod fillets (4 @ .33 lb. ea.)
- 6 minced garlic cloves (6)

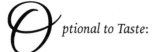

ptional to Taste:

- Garlic powder
- Salt

H ow To Prepare:

1. Melt the ghee and about half of the garlic into a skillet.
2. Arrange the fillets in the pan using the medium-high heat

setting. Sprinkle with the garlic powder, pepper, and the salt.

3. Once it turns white halfway up its side, turn it over, and add the remainder of the minced garlic. Continue cooking until it flakes easily.

4. Serve with some ghee-garlic from the pan.

 ork-Chop Fat Bombs

 ervings: 3

Total Macro Nutrients:

- 7 g Net Carbs
- 30 g Total Protein
- 103 g Total Fats
- 1076 Calories

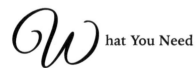 hat You Need

- Boneless pork chops (3)
- Oil (.5 cup)
- Medium yellow onion (1)
- Brown mushrooms (8 oz.)
- Nutmeg (1 tsp.)
- Garlic powder (1 tsp.)
- Balsamic vinegar (1 tbsp.)
- Mayonnaise (1 cup)

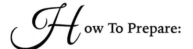

How To Prepare:

1. Rinse, drain, and slice the mushrooms. Peel and slice the onion. Put them in a large skillet with the oil and sauté until wilted.
2. Place the chops to the side and sprinkle with the nutmeg and garlic powder. Cook until done. Transfer the prepared chops onto a plate.
3. Whisk in the vinegar and mayonnaise into the pan. The thick sauce can be thinned with a bit of chicken broth if needed. (Add 2 tablespoons at a time.)
4. Ladle the sauce over the bomb and serve.

Pork Kebabs

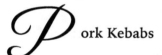

Servings: 4

Total Macro Nutrients:

- 3.3 g Net Carbs
- 33.7 g Total Protein
- 8.6 g Total Fats

What You Need:

- Hot sauce (2 tsp.)
- Sunflower seed butter (3 tbsp.)
- Minced garlic (1 tbsp.)
- Keto-friendly soy sauce (1 tbsp.)
- Water (1 tbsp.)
- Medium green pepper (1)
- Crushed red pepper (.5 tsp.)
- Squared pork for kebabs (1 lb.)

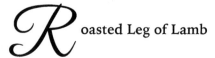

How to Prepare:

1. Warm up the oven or grill using the broil or the high heat setting.
2. In a processor or blender, combine the water with the red pepper, soy sauce, garlic, butter, and hot sauce.
3. Slice the pork into squares. Cover with the marinade and rest for one hour.
4. Chop the peppers to fit the skewer. Thread the skewers alternating the pork and peppers.
5. Broil using the high heat setting for five minutes per side.

Roasted Leg of Lamb

Servings: 2

Total Macro Nutrients:

- 1 g Net Carbs

- 22 g Total Protein
- 14 g Total Fats
- 223 Calories

*W*hat You Need:

- Reduced-sodium beef broth (.5 cup)
- Leg of lamb (2 lb.)
- Chopped garlic cloves (6)
- Fresh rosemary leaves (1 tbsp.)
- Black pepper (1 tsp.)
- Salt (2 tsp.)

*H*ow To Prepare:

1. Grease a baking pan and set the oven temperature to 400° Fahrenheit.
2. Arrange the lamb in the pan and add the broth and seasonings.
3. Roast 30 minutes and lower the heat to 350° Fahrenheit. Continue cooking for about one hour or until done.
4. Let the lamb stand about 20 minutes before slicing to serve.
5. Enjoy with some roasted Brussels sprouts and extra rosemary for a tasty change of pace.

Slow-Cooked London Broil

Servings: 4

Total Macro Nutrients:

- 2.6 g Net Carbs
- 47.3 g Total Protein
- 18.3 g Total Fats
- 409 Calories

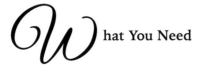

What You Need

- London broil (2 lb.)
- Dijon mustard (1 tbsp.)
- Reduced sugar ketchup (2 tbsp.)
- Coconut Aminos or your favorite soy sauce substitute (2 tbsp.)
- Coffee (.5 cup)
- Chicken broth (.5 cup)
- White wine (.25 cup)
- Onion powder (2 tsp.)
- Minced garlic (2 tsp.)

How To Prepare:

1. Arrange the beef in the cooker. Cover both sides with the mustard, soy sauce, ketchup, and minced garlic.
2. Pour the liquids into the cooker and give it a sprinkle of the onion powder.
3. Cook for four to six hours. When the timer buzzes, shred the meat. Combine with the juices and serve.

Stuffed Pork Tenderloin

Servings: 6

Total Macro Nutrients:

- 2.9 g Net Carbs
- 28.8 g Total Protein
- 6.2 g Total Fats
- 194 Calories

What You Need:

- Pork tenderloin or venison (2 lb.)
- Feta cheese (.5 cup)
- Gorgonzola cheese (.5 cup)
- Chopped onion (1 tsp.)

- Minced garlic (2 cloves)
- Crushed almonds (2 tbsp.)
- Sea Salt & black pepper (.5 tsp. each)

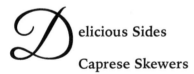 ow To Prepare:

1. Warm up the grill. Create a pocket in the tenderloin using a sharp knife.
2. Combine the cheeses, onions, almonds, and garlic.
3. Stuff the pork pocket and seal using a skewer.
4. Grill until done with the lid closed (about 300-350° Fahrenheit). The center of the meat should reach 150° Fahrenheit.)
5. Let it rest about 15 minutes tented with foil before serving.

*D*elicious Sides

Caprese Skewers

*S*ervings: 2

Total Macro Nutrients:

- 7 g Net Carbs
- 24.5 g Total Protein
- 27.4 g Total Fats
- 384 Calories

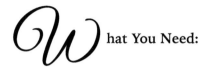

hat You Need:

- Baby mozzarella cheese balls (2 cups)
- Cherry or baby heirloom tomatoes (2 cups)
- Pitted mixed olives (.5 cup)
- Green/red pesto (2 tbsp.)
- Fresh basil (2 tbsp.)

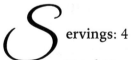

ow To Prepare:

1. Rinse the basil and tomatoes.
2. Marinate the kalamata and green olives in extra-virgin olive oil with the oregano.
3. Combine the mozzarella with the pesto.
4. Arrange the olives, mozzarella, and tomatoes onto the skewers and garnish with the basil.
5. Serve any time.

Mock Mac 'N' Cheese

ervings: 4

Total Macro Nutrients:

- 7 g Net Carbs
- 11 g Total Protein
- 23 g Total Fats

- 294 Calories

*W*hat You Need:

- Cauliflower (1 head)
- Butter (3 tbsp.)
- Unsweetened almond milk (.25 cup)
- Heavy cream (.25 cup)
- Cheddar cheese (1 cup)
- Freshly cracked black pepper & Sea salt (as desired)

*H*ow To Prepare:

1. Use a sharp knife to slice the cauliflower into small florets. Shred the cheese.
2. Prepare the oven to reach 450° Fahrenheit. Cover a baking sheet with a layer of parchment paper or foil.
3. Melt 2 tbsp. of the butter in a saucepan. Toss the florets and butter together. Sprinkle with the pepper and salt. Place the cauliflower on the baking pan and roast 10-15 minutes.
4. Warm up the rest of the butter, milk, heavy cream, and cheese in the microwave or double boiler. Pour the cheese over the cauliflower and serve.

Parmesan Onion Rings

Servings: 4

Total Macro Nutrients:

- 5 g Net Carbs
- 3 g Total Protein
- 7 g Total Fats
- 89 Calories

What You Need:

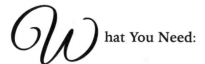

- Large white onion (1)
- Medium egg (1)
- Pepper to taste
- Parmesan cheese (1 tbsp.)
- Coconut flour (1 tbsp.)
- Heavy cream (1 tbsp.)
- Olive oil – for frying

How To Prepare:

1. In a skillet, warm the oil until it reaches 350° Fahrenheit.
2. Slice the onions into thick rings.

3. Whisk the flour, cheese, and pepper.

4. Whisk the cream and egg together.

5. Dip the sliced rings into the wet and then the dry mixture. Gently add to the oil. Cook for two to three minutes. Drain on a towel-lined platter. Serve while hot.

Roasted Veggies

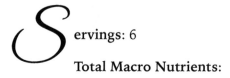

Servings: 6

Total Macro Nutrients:

- 3 g Net Carbs
- 2 g Total Protein
- 5 g Total Fats
- 65 Calories

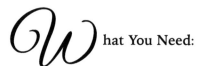

What You Need:

- Button mushrooms (1 cup)
- Sliced zucchini (2)
- Large grape tomatoes (8)
- Chopped asparagus spears (10)
- Chopped yellow pepper (1)
- Olive oil (2 tbsp.)
- Freshly squeezed lemon juice (1 tbsp.)
- Salt (.5 tsp.)

How To Prepare:

1. Prepare the oven to 450° Fahrenheit. Lightly grease a baking pan.
2. Slice and chop the veggies. Place them into the prepared pan.
3. Toss gently with the oil and juice. Sprinkle with the salt and roast 40 minutes. Stir every 10 minutes to prevent sticking and allow even cooking.

DELICIOUS SNACKS & DESSERTS

ALMOND CREAMY & Dark Chocolate Bombs

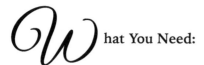ervings: 12

Total Macro Nutrients:

- 2 g Net Carbs
- 2 g Total Protein
- 7 g Total Fats
- 86 Calories

hat You Need:

- Regular cream cheese (1 oz.)
- Coconut butter - not oil (4 tbsp.)

- Almond butter (4 tbsp.)
- 73% organic super dark chocolate - 2 sections
- Sugar-free French vanilla syrup (2 tbsp.)
- Cocoa powder - unsweetened (1 tbsp.)
- Optional: 2 packets of stevia/sweetener of choice

ow To Prepare:

1. In a microwavable dish, add all fixings except the coconut butter.
2. Cook at 15-second intervals until the chocolate has melted. Stir all ingredients until incorporated.
3. Spoon the batter into 12 muffin tins or use silicone candy molds.
4. Place the container of bombs in the freezer for about one hour.
5. Just quickly pop them out using a butter knife. Store and enjoy!

acon Guacamole Fat Bombs

Servings: 6

Total Macro Nutrients:

- 1.4 g Net Carbs
- 3.4 g Total Protein
- 15.2 g Total Fats

- 156 Calories

*W*hat You Need

- Avocado (3.5 oz. or about .5 of 1 large)
- Bacon (about 4 oz. - 4 strips)
- Ghee or butter (.25 cup)
- Crushed cloves of garlic (2)
- Small diced onion (approximately 1.2 oz. or .5 of 1)
- Small finely chopped chili pepper (1)
- Fresh lime juice (1 tbsp. or about .25 of a lime)
- Pinch of ground black pepper or cayenne (1 pinch)
- Salt (to your liking)
- Freshly chopped cilantro (1-2 tbsp.)

*H*ow To Prepare:

1. Heat up the oven temperature to 375° Fahrenheit. Prepare a baking tray with parchment paper and cook the bacon for 10 to 15 minutes. Save the grease for step four.
2. Peel, deseed, and chop the avocado into a dish along with the garlic, chili pepper, lime juice, cilantro, black pepper, salt, and butter. Use a fork or potato masher to combine the mixture. Blend in the onion.
3. Empty the grease into the bomb fixings, blend well, and cover for 20 to 30 minutes in the fridge.

4. Break up the bacon into a bowl and roll the six balls in it until coated evenly. Serve or eat when you want a delicious snack.

acon Wrapped Mozzarella Sticks

ervings: 2

Total Macro Nutrients:

- 1 g Net Carbs
- 7 g Total Protein
- 9 g Total Fats
- 103 Calories

hat You Need:

- Thick bacon (2 slices)
- Frigo cheese head mozzarella cheese sticks (1)
- Coconut oil – for frying

hat You Need For Optional Dipping:

- Low-sugar pizza sauce

- Toothpicks

How To Prepare:

1. Warm up the oil to 350° Fahrenheit in a deep fryer.
2. Slice the cheese stick in half. Wrap it with the bacon and secure it closed using the toothpick.
3. Cook the sticks in the hot fryer for 2-3 minutes.
4. Drain on a towel and cool. Serve with your sauce.

Chocolate Chip Cookie Dough Fat Bomb

Servings: 20

Total Macro Nutrients:

- 2 g Net Carbs
- 2 g Total Protein
- 14 g Total Fats
- 139 Calories

What You Need:

- Cream cheese (1 pkg. - 8 oz.)

- Salted butter (.5 cup or 1 stick)
- Sweetener – swerve/erythritol (.33 cup)
- Almond butter or creamy peanut butter - only salt and peanuts (.5 cup)
- Vanilla extract (1 tsp.)
- Baking chips - stevia sweetened chocolate chips (4 oz.)

*H*ow To Prepare:

1. Remove the cream cheese from the fridge for about 20 to 30 minutes to soften.
2. Use a mixer to blend all of the fixings. Refrigerate at least 30 minutes before adding them onto a tray lined with a layer of parchment paper.
3. Spray an ice cream scoop with a spritz of cooking spray (preferably coconut oil).
4. Scoop out 20 bomb portions and place them onto the prepared pan.
5. Freeze for a minimum of 30 minutes.
6. Store in the fridge in a zipper-type plastic bag for convenience.

*K*ale Chips

*S*ervings: 2

Total Macro Nutrients:

- 0.5 g Net Carbs
- 4 g Total Protein
- 8 g Total Fats
- 180 Calories

What You Need:

- Kale (1 bunch)
- Crushed red pepper (1 tsp.)
- Garlic powder (1 tsp.)
- Olive oil (2 tbsp.)
- Parmesan cheese (2 tbsp.)

How To Prepare:

1. Program the oven setting until it reaches 350° Fahrenheit.
2. Rinse and dry the kale. Tear it into pieces.
3. Pour the oil over the pieces and toss to combine. Evenly arrange the kale on a baking tin.
4. Bake for 8 minutes. If they are not done, continue baking, checking at 2-minute intervals (approximately 12 min. should be okay).
5. Cool them down for several minutes. Serve when they're crunchy the way you like them.

Desserts

Blackberry Almond Chia Pudding

. . .

*S*ervings: 2

Total Macro Nutrients:

- 1 g Net Carbs
- 2 g Total Protein
- 8 g Total Fats
- 109 Calories

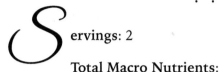*W*hat You Need:

- Chia seeds (.25 cup)
- Raw honey (drizzle)
- Sliced almonds (2-3 tbsp.)
- Vanilla almond milk (1.5 cups)
- Fresh blackberries (6 oz.)

*H*ow To Prepare:

1. Rinse and add the berries into a dish. Crush with a fork until creamy.
2. Pour in the raw honey, milk, and chia seeds. Stir well.
3. Refrigerate for several hours or overnight for the most delicious results.
4. Sprinkle with the almonds and several blackberries.
5. Serve any time.

o-Bake Chocolate Peanut Butter Fat Bombs

 ervings: 8

Total Macro Nutrients:

- 0.8 g Net Carbs
- 4.4 g Total Protein
- 20 g Total Fats
- 208 Calories

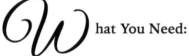 hat You Need:

- Shelled hemp seeds (6 tbsp.)
- PB Fit Powder (4 tbsp.)
- Coconut oil (.5 cup)
- Heavy cream (2 tbsp.)
- Cocoa powder (.25 cup)
- Unsweetened shredded coconut (.25 cup)
- Liquid stevia (28 drops)
- Vanilla extract (1 tsp.)

H ow To Prepare:

1. Combine all of the dry fixings and blend in the oil which will create a paste.
2. Mix the heavy cream, stevia, and vanilla into the paste - until just combined. Shape into eight balls.
3. Dump the coconut on a flat surface. Roll the balls through it.
4. Arrange the balls in a dish. Store in the freezer compartment for a minimum of 20 minutes.

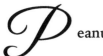 eanut Butter Fudge

 ervings: 18

Total Macro Nutrients:

- -0- g Net Carbs
- 2 g Total Protein
- 8 g Total Fats
- 89 Calories

 hat You Need:

- Coconut oil (.5 cup)
- Peanut butter (.5 cup)
- Liquid stevia granulated sweetener (as desired)
- Also Needed: 12-18 count muffin tin & liners or a loaf pan

ow To Prepare:

1. Prepare the tin of choice with a spritz of oil.
2. Combine the oil and peanut butter together on the stovetop or microwave. Melt and add the sweetener.
3. Scoop into the tins or loaf pan and freeze.
4. You can serve with a drizzle of melted chocolate – but remember to count the carbs.

 ## eanut Butter Protein Bars

 ## ervings: 12

Total Macro Nutrients:

- 3 g Net Carbs
- 7 g Total Protein
- 14 g Total Fats
- 172 Calories

hat You Need:

- Almond meal (1.5 cups)
- Keto-friendly chunky peanut butter (1 cup)
- Egg whites (2)
- Almonds (.5 cup)

- Cashews (.5 cup)
- Also Needed: Baking pan

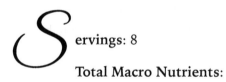

*H*ow To Prepare:

1. Heat the oven ahead of time to reach 350° Fahrenheit.
2. Spritz a baking dish lightly with coconut or olive oil.
3. Combine all of the fixings and add to the prepared dish.
4. Bake for 15 minutes and cut into 12 pieces once they're cooled.
5. Store in the refrigerator to keep them fresh.

Pumpkin Bread

*S*ervings: 8

Total Macro Nutrients:

- 5 g Net Carbs
- 8 g Total Protein
- 26 g Total Fats
- 311 Calories

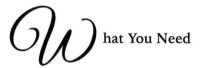

*W*hat You Need

- Almond flour (1 cup)
- Libby's Canned Pumpkin (1 small can)

- Baking powder (.5 tsp.)
- Coconut flour (.5 cup)
- Heavy cream (.5 cup)
- Stevia (.5 cup)
- Melted butter (1 stick)
- Large eggs (4)
- Vanilla (1.5 tsp.)
- Pumpkin spice (2 tsp.)

How To Prepare:

1. Set the oven temperature setting to 350° Fahrenheit. Grease a pie plate with a spritz of coconut oil.
2. Combine all of the fixings in a mixing container until light and fluffy.
3. Pour the batter into the prepared pan. Bake for approximately 70 to 90 minutes.

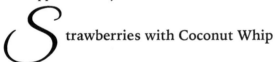 Strawberries with Coconut Whip

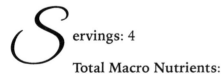 Servings: 4

Total Macro Nutrients:

- 10 g Net Carbs
- 4 g Total Protein
- 31 g Total Fats
- 342 Calories

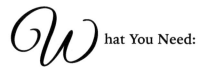

What You Need:

- Strawberries or other favorite berries (4 cups)
- Refrigerated coconut cream (2 cans)
- Unsweetened chopped dark chocolate - 70% or darker (1 oz.)

How To Prepare:

1. Remove the solidified cream from the can of milk and set aside for another time, saving the liquid. Pour it into a mixing container and whip with a hand mixer until it forms stiff peaks (approximately five minutes).
2. Slice the berries and portion into four dishes. Serve with a dollop of the cream. Garnish with the chopped chocolate and a few berries. Serve.

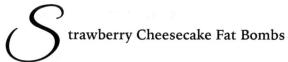

Strawberry Cheesecake Fat Bombs

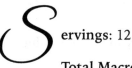

Servings: 12

Total Macro Nutrients:

- 0.85 g Net Carbs

- 0.96 g Total Protein
- 7.4 g Total Fats
- 67 Calories

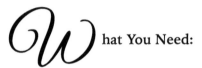 hat You Need:

- Coconut oil or softened butter (.25 cup)
- Softened cream cheese (.75 cup)
- Fresh/frozen strawberries (.5 cup)
- Liquid stevia (10-15 drops) or powdered erythritol (2 tbsp.)
- Vanilla extract (1 tbsp.)

ℋ ow To Prepare:

1. Mix the butter or coconut oil with the cream cheese in a mixing container. Let it rest 30-60 minutes until it is room temperature. (Don't microwave.)
2. Prepare the berries and remove the stems. Add them to a dish and mash until smooth. Stir in the stevia and vanilla. Mix well using a food processor or hand whisk.
3. Scoop out the mixture and add into candy molds or muffin silicone molds.
4. Let the bombs rest in the freezer until set, usually about two hours.
5. Just pop them out and enjoy. Store in the freezer.

Strawberry Thumbprint Delights

Servings: 16

Total Macro Nutrients:

- 1 g Net Carbs
- 2 g Total Protein
- 9 g Total Fats
- 95 Calories

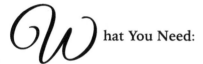

What You Need:

- Almond flour (1 cup)
- Baking powder (.5 tsp.)
- Coconut flour (2 tbsp.)
- Sugar-free strawberry jam (2 tbsp.)
- Shredded coconut (1 tbsp.)
- Eggs (2)
- Erythritol (.5 cup)
- Coconut oil (4 tbsp.)
- Salt (.5 tsp.)
- Cinnamon (.5 tsp.)
- Almond extract (.5 tsp.)
- Vanilla extract (.5 tsp.)

*H*ow To Prepare:

1. Warm up the oven temperature to 350° Fahrenheit. Cover a cookie tin with a sheet of parchment paper.
2. Whisk the dry fixings and make a hole in the middle. Fold in the wet fixings to form a dough. Break it into 16 segments and roll into balls.
3. Arrange each one on the prepared cookie sheet and bake 15 minutes.
4. When done, cool completely and add a dab of jam to each one with a sprinkle of coconut.

CONCLUSION

I sincerely hope that you enjoyed each segment of the *Intermittent Fasting: A Guide to Burn Fat, Weight Loss, Improve Health, Healing – Low Carb Keto Diet Recipes*. I hope it was informative and provided you with all of the tools you need to achieve your goals of losing weight and to become healthier. As you read through your new book, many simple tips were provided for your ketogenic journey. These are just several of them, so you have them fresh in your mind:

- Drink plenty of water daily and limit the intake of sugar-sweetened beverages.
- Use only fat-free or low-fat condiments.
- Read the food labels and make choices that keep you in line with ketosis.
- Add a serving of vegetables to your dinner and lunch menus.
- For a snack, have some frozen yogurt (fat-free or low-fat), nuts or unsalted pretzels, raw veggies, or unsalted-plain popcorn.

One last recipe for success:

Bone Broth

This remedy has been around for many years. The broth can eliminate keto flu symptoms and provide you with an increase of your essential electrolytes. The broth can boost your immune system, help keep your intestinal tract healthier, and increase collagen levels to improve your eyes, heart, skin, joints, and bones. You will also achieve improved brain health.

Make yourself a batch anytime to sip or use in your cooking. Use the recipe below:

Servings: 6-8 cups

Total Macro Nutrients:

- 0.7 g Net Carbs
- 3.6 g Total Protein
- 6 g Total Fats
- 72 Calories

What You Need

- Mixed assorted bones – ex. marrow bones, chicken feet, pork or your choice (3.5 lb.)
- Pink Himalayan salt (1 tbsp.)
- Medium parsnip (1)
- Medium white onion – skin on (1)
- Minced garlic (5 cloves)
- Medium celery (2 stalks)
- Medium Carrots (2)
- Apple cider vinegar or lemon juice (2 tbsp.)
- Water (8 cups)

- Also Needed: Slow cooker

How To Prepare:

1. Peel and slice the vegetables with roots into 1/3-inch pieces. Slice the onion in half. Chop the celery into thirds. Add the bay leaves into the slow cooker.
2. Toss in the chosen bones. Pour the water up to ¾ capacity – along with the juice/vinegar, and bay leaves. Sprinkle with the salt.
3. Secure the lid. Choose either low (ten hours) or high (six hours). You can simmer up to 48 hours.
4. Use a strainer to remove the bits of veggies. Set the bones aside to chill. Shred the meat and use as desired.
5. Refrigerate the broth overnight. Scrape away the tallow (greasy layer) if desired. Use within five days or freeze. You can also keep it in the canning jars for up to 45 days.

By now, you have decided which of the intermittent fasting techniques you will be using on this journey. Try one of the plans and give it some time for your body to adjust. This is not a miracle diet but a new way of living. You also know how you can best mix and match to find the perfect solution for you. Making the decision to alter your original eating patterns is a major one, and it is crucial that you take the full weight of the decision into account before acting.

If you are convinced that you have what it takes to take full advantage of the benefits that intermittent fasting has to offer, then the next step is to stop reading and to start fasting. Choose the type of intermittent fasting technique that seems like the best fit for you and give it a try. You have a plentiful supply of recipes to use to begin the program.

Try not to become discouraged if you don't receive immediate results. Make an effort to find the one that's right for you. Above all, don't rush, and remember, intermittent fasting is a marathon not a sprint, slow and steady will win the race.

Finally, if you found this book useful in any way, a review on Amazon is always appreciated!

INDEX

Smoothies

INDEX

- *Blueberry Essence*
- *Mocha 5-Minute Smoothie*

VEGAN
MEAL PREP

30-Day Meal Plan – Easy Recipes for Weight Loss, Busy People & Healthy Living

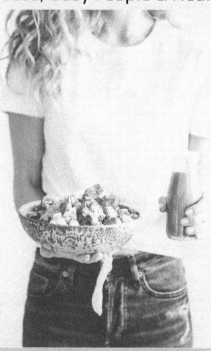

Elyse Bose

WHAT IS VEGANISM?

THINK of the first thing that comes to your mind when you hear the term "vegan." You might think about Instagram, you might think about Netflix food documentaries, or you might think about the global environmental crisis. While none of these are necessarily the wrong ways to think about veganism, there are lots of misconceptions about what it means to live a vegan lifestyle. There are many different definitions of being a "vegan," but regardless of which one you choose, veganism affects more than just your diet. Animal products are everywhere, and if you commit to being entirely vegan, you're going to need to take a hard look at the way you live your life. While you don't have to subscribe to every belief about veganism, you'll want to make sure to pay extra attention to your sauces and the ingredients in foods you haven't cooked yourself – which can be time-consuming. But animal products are often hidden in bready pastries, fruit smoothies, and other foods you wouldn't expect to contain them. Meat is easy to spot, but the health of a vegan diet goes deeper than simply choosing a vegetable over a steak. Regardless of how you practice your veganism, however, there is absolutely no scientific dispute over the incredible health benefits a vegan diet has for human beings. Vegetables, fruits, nuts, beans, and seeds offer way more nutritional value per gram of sustenance than meat products, dairy, and processed grains. A vegan diet supplies your body with the most nutritional and valuable possible nutrients straight from the source, where most meat eaters would lose out. Animals eat plants, but when we eat animals, the nutrients we get from the plants are so far removed, they make little to no difference. Eating plants fresh instead of indirectly cuts out the middle man, which is especially beneficial if the middle man is pumped full of hormones, steroids, and antibiotics. Speaking of animal hormone therapy, let's talk a little bit more in-depth about why exactly animal products are so bad for us, and for our planet before we get into the exciting details of how a vegan diet can help you lose that stubborn weight that's been holding you down.

Animals and Our Environment

Veganism is probably most famous for its stance against the cruel treatment of animals in the farming industry that drives vegans not to eat meat. You don't have to be an animal rights activist to want to encourage the more humane treatment of our fellow species, but you also don't have to be an animal rights activist to know that the chemicals that meat is treated with aren't healthy. However, that's a topic we'll cover more in-depth late in this chapter. For now, veganism makes an important impact on the environment that you should also be aware of – because of your efforts to make a difference. The farming industry requires billions of dollars per year just to sustain itself, and that isn't including the cost of packaging after the animal products are ready to be sealed and shipped out. Raising an animal just to use it as a food source means that the farming industry consumes almost as much plant material and water to feed the animals as we could be eating ourselves as humans. Not to mention that by the time the nutrients in the plants have been digested and absorbed by the animal, they'll likely be of little use to us when we consume that same animal. So why are we even feeding valuable and nutritional material to animals who are simply going to make us unhealthier when we consume them? There's a key economic component at play within the food industry that affects the accessibility of meats and vegetables, and it's a fairly big deal: meat is simply cheaper. Food for livestock is under government subsidy in many high-producing countries, which means that farmers have to pay less to produce more product. Unfortunately, that fact becomes catastrophic when you discover that in the United States alone, fourteen times the amount of farmland is used to raise plants and vegetables for livestock feed that is allocated for edible produce. More clearly, that means that only one-fourteenth of the agricultural land in the United States grows produce meant for humans to eat. World hunger suddenly seems a bit more sinister when you understand the amount of wasted material that goes towards raising an animal for consumption. And that's not to mention that meat is also easier to store and ship since it won't go rotten as quickly as vegetables. All of these factors contribute to an industry that's wasting a decent amount of our natural resources trying to sustain an unsustainable source.

Veganism and Losing Weight

The honest truth about a vegan diet is that you don't even have to eat an evenly balanced, truly healthy vegan diet in order to lose weight. The amount of processing that occurs in the food packaging industry when it comes to animal products adds so many unhealthy chemicals and makes so many unhealthy changes to your natural ingredients that even a small portion of crispy fried vegetables will make a difference in your weight. However, with a fully realized vegan diet, you'll be cutting out so many heavy saturated fats that even without a strict workout regime, your body will burn fatter because your metabolism will be higher. We'll take a closer look at this miraculous metabolism boost in the next section, but another key factor that veganism contributes to weight loss is fiber. The large majority of American adults don't get enough fiber in their diets because the best sources of fiber are fruits and vegetables. You've probably seen the various chocolate chip-filled fiber bars at the grocery store marketed towards individuals with poor diets – but vegetables are a much healthier source. Fiber is crucial for healthy digestion, but it's also an important regulatory mechanism for your blood sugar. Fiber is tough and difficult for our system to digest, and so, it tends to take much longer to move through your digestive system. When digestion occurs too quickly, as it often does with processed foods that are flimsy and lack nutrition, your intestines absorb sugar too quickly and your blood sugar spikes. When you digest fiber, the longer time it takes to move through your digestive tract, the longer time your body has to slowly and properly absorb the nutrients and sugars into your bloodstream. Instead of spiking your blood sugar just to crash it later, fiber raises your blood sugar slowly and safely and allows your body to maintain homeostasis. Without fiber, you're also more likely to have irregular bowel movements that will further prevent your digestive tract from properly absorbing nutrients. Fiber has many other tentative benefits that haven't been corroborated by science, but as with most lifestyle changes during a vegan diet, there can come nothing but good health and weight loss when you replace artificial ingredients with fresh, natural sources.

. . .

*H*ow Veggies Keep You Healthy

Now that you understand how veganism can help you lose weight, let's learn from metabolism and vegetables about what's really going to happen to your body when you go vegan. The science behind eating a vegan diet is incredibly simple and also incredibly confusing when you finally understand and wonder why more people don't choose to eat vegan. We'll start from the very basic and work our way up. Nutritious food is nutritious because it offers our bodies something we need. But we don't just need one thing. There is a vast stable of vitamins, minerals, fats, proteins, and carbohydrates that we need in our diet for our body to be able to perform our various life functions. When you add all of these so-called "life functions" together, processes like digestion, circulation, and muscle growth, you get what's called your metabolism. That's right – if you thought your metabolism was only how effectively your body digested and used nutrients, you missed a few more important details. Your metabolism is basically a measure of how effectively your body is able to sustain your body, so it goes to follow that if you aren't fuelling up on the proper sources, you won't be able to sustain a high metabolism. There are certain unhealthy foods that contribute more seriously than others to damaging our metabolisms. Although you're most likely tempted to say that fats and oils are the biggest culprits of an unhealthy diet, that's not always the case. And neither is your second option, sugar – glucose is actually your body's preferred source of energy. So how can these foods be bad for us, if they're exactly what our body needs?

. . .

*T*he biggest culprits of modern unhealthy food production and consumption happen to be ourselves. In the late nineteen-seventies, large-scale farming and packaging operations began to implement a process called "hydrogenation" in their sealing and shipping regimes. Hydrogenation hardens the soft, whole fats and oils that are naturally found in foods so that their consistency is more solid. Foods containing hydrogenated fats and oils won't go bad as quickly as they would have, had they *not* been hydrogenized. Which doesn't seem quite right straight out of the gate - but there's more. Hydrogenated fats and oils, also known as saturated fats or trans fats, are incredibly bad for us. They raise our levels of bad cholesterol and lower our levels of good cholesterol. (If you didn't already know, now you do – cholesterol isn't just a number. It's a type of molecule, and we need the good version to help facilitate passage through our cell walls, create important enzymes for digestion, and build hormones. Bad cholesterol is what causes your doctor to warn you about arterial plaque if your good cholesterol numbers aren't looking great. Bad cholesterol is found in all saturated fats and oils, and it's the nasty molecule that causes plaque to build up in the arteries around your heart. When plaque builds up inside an artery, the arterial pressure at that point of your heart will skyrocket. In order to compensate for the blockage, your heart muscles have to pump harder and harder to move the same amount of blood. Atherosclerosis comes hand-in-hand with bad cholesterol, and if this swelling of the heart muscles starts to happen to you, you're at risk for a heart attack.

*B*ut what do these saturated fats and oils have to do with eating a vegan diet? Remember back to before the fats and oils from earlier were hydrogenized. They were perfectly healthy. Whole fats and natural sugars that are good for us? When fats and oils occur in nature, they're amazing for us. We need whole fats and natural oils to properly dissolve vitamins, synthesize hormones, and make new cells. In fact, it's physically impossible for your body to digest Vitamin E, Vitamin D, Vitamin K, and Vitamin A without fat molecules present. Dairy products are packed with fat, but think about the last time you consumed a dairy product that wasn't in some way processed or packaged. Dairy products go through a myriad of different artificial processes to keep them from going bad. More processes, in fact, than any other food group – including vegetables. What might've been good for us at one time is now packed full of unhealthy and dangerous fat molecules. The more time you spend eating vegetables and fruits, cooking your own meals instead of eating out, and skipping on the packaged and processed goods, the more time you'll tack on to the end of your life.

SUPPLEMENTING YOUR VEGAN LIFESTYLE

NOT ALL VEGANS feel the need to take supplements, but when it comes down to the science of supplementing your diet with vitamins and minerals that you're most likely missing, even non-vegans should consider supplements. However, for your specific vegan lifestyle, it's important to realize that unless you've spent an impressive amount of time studying the food pyramid and portion sizes, it's very easy to be deficient. Most individuals eating a regular, full-fat, full-meat diet today have deficiencies in iron, vitamin D, calcium, and vitamin B12. Although these deficiencies do tend to vary slightly by country and region, a shocking number of people are still missing them. In your vegan diet particularly, you'll find that you need more calcium and iron, as well as an Omega-3 supplement and a zinc supplement. Omega-3 is found mainly in fish and fish oil, so if you aren't comfortable consuming an oil that's still technically an animal product, try switching it out with flaxseed oil or canola oil (bonus tip: canola oil is even lower in calories and fat content than olive oil, so if you're not looking for a particularly olive-flavored dish, swap them out!). Vegans should also take an iodine supplement. Iodine is found mainly in seafood, but it is essential for creating hormones for your thyroid gland. While you can rely on a multi-vitamin to give you enough iodine, a multi-vitamin likely won't give you enough of any of the above vitamins and minerals to justify taking one by itself. You should always buy your supplements in bulk and in individually measured tablets so that you can control your dosages. Keep in mind, though, as you consider which supplements you're going to take – there's plenty of scientific research on alternative ways to supply yourself with some of these vitamins and minerals, but it's likely that you won't be able to get a large enough dosage. Plants, nuts, seeds, and legumes are all packed with some of the vitamins and minerals you'll be taking, but their percentages are small, and you can't always be accurate based on portions. Taking too many vitamins luckily doesn't do you any harm, so it's really in your best interest to consider what a supplement might offer your vegan diet.

What Vegan Portions Should Look Like

A vegan diet should always be a balance between all-natural vegetable-based proteins, carbohydrates, and fats, with little room for added sugars and no room for animal products. But carbohydrates aren't as healthy as fruits and vegetables, and eating too much protein doesn't actually help your diet. As a vegan, it is just as important to know the amounts of what you'll be eating as it is to know where the ingredients came from. In order to eat a vegan diet that also facilitates weight loss in combination with your workout routine, you should portion out your meals based on weight and nutrients. In order to determine how many, and of what type of nutrients are in your vegan meals, let's take a look at some more nutritional science and learn about two sections of your diet that you wouldn't be able to live without.

· · ·
$\mathcal{M}$acros and Micros

If you're not overly familiar with the bodybuilding world, you might not have ever heard of "macros" and "micros." In a more familiar terminology, "macros" stands for "macronutrients," and you can guess that "micros" stands for "micronutrients."As we've been discussing the various sources of fuel that your body relies on to function, we've been focused mostly on macronutrients. These are the most important three categories of nutrients that your body relies on the most heavily. You know them as carbohydrates, proteins, and fats! Suddenly, it doesn't seem too intimidating to "track your macros", if tracking you macros simply means making sure you're eating a balanced portion of each of these categories. Especially as a vegan, you're going to be much more likely to receive a higher amount of macronutrients in your diet – just by virtue of eating more fruits and vegetables. However, just like everything else in our bodies, our macronutrients still need to be balanced. A diet that's too high in carbohydrates is going to be packed with sugars, and if you don't live a high-intensity active lifestyle, this type of macronutrient imbalance will make you gain weight. Don't be intimidated though – it's very easy as a vegan to track your macros and make sure you're not eating too many of one category. This is also another reason prepping your meals is so important: you'll get to see a visual representation of how many of each macronutrient you're consuming during each meal. The most realistic distribution of macronutrients for a vegan looks something like 1/5 protein, 3/5 carbohydrates, and 2/5 fats. There are plenty of great online resources that have macronutrient calculators, but before you can learn how to track your macros, you'll need to learn what "micros" are, and how a food scale is about to become your most important tool for vegan weight loss and meal prep.

Understanding Micronutrients

While your macronutrients tend to be the larger groups of food you're consuming while eating a vegan diet, your *micronutrients* (the abbreviation "micros" makes sense now!) are those trickier-to-get vitamins and minerals that you can't always consume enough of. There is often no way of knowing just what the micronutrient content is of certain plants and fruits, although we are able to tell that citrus fruits contain Vitamin C, carrots contain Vitamin A, and chia seeds contain calcium. Think back to what you learned about supplementing your vegan diet with vitamins and minerals. These important micronutrients don't just help your body run its own life processes; vitamins and minerals are essential for aiding macronutrients in *their* important work raising your good cholesterol, synthesizing new proteins, and fueling your brain.

Vitamins and minerals can't hurt you if you take too many, but think about the impact it could have on your metabolism and lifetime health if your body isn't getting a good supply of either macronutrients or micronutrients. Because of the way the food industry packages and present our meals, we often hear more about sugar content, saturated and trans fats, and sodium content. Although it's great to know when any one of those ingredients is present in our food, they're all still ingredients that are bad for us. Further down nutritional labels, you can often find vitamin contents and a few mineral additions here and there, but these are the ingredient we should be so focused on and not the negative ones.

*O*ne of the benefits of meal prepping is that you get to control your nutrition at its most basic level, so you can watch and determine just how many of each macro and micronutrient your body gets. This authority alone will immediately help you lose weight, as your body adjusts to running at maximum function off a healthy and sustainable natural diet. That begs the question, however – when you're meal prepping at home, how exactly *do* you make sure that you're getting your proper distribution of nutrients? If your scale isn't your best friend these days, get ready to meet a new type of weighing device that's going to help you fall in love with you waistline all over again.

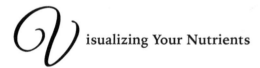 isualizing Your Nutrients

DAILY REQUIRED NUTRIENTS

LOW ACTIVITY

Carbohydrate 65% - Protien 15% - Fat 20%

MEDIUM ACTIVITY

Carbohydrate 60% - Protien 20% - Fat 20%

HIGH ACTIVITY

Carbohydrate 55% - Protien 25% - Fat 20%

DAILY REQUIRED MICRONUTRIENTS

Vitamin A 5,000 IU

Vitamin B6 2 mg

Vitamin B12 6 micrograms

Vitamin C 60 mg

Vitamin D 400 IU

Vitamin E 80 micrograms

Vitamin K 80 micrograms

Calcium 1000 mg

Biotin 300 micrograms

Chloride 3400 micrograms

Chromium 120 micrograms

Copper 2 mg

Folate 400 micrograms

Iron 18 mg

Iodine 150 micrograms

Magnesium 400 micrograms

Manganese 2 mg

Molybdenum 75 micrograms

Niacin 20 mg

Pantothenic Acid 10 mg

Phosphorus 1000 mg

Riboflavin 1.7 mg

Selenium 70 micrograms

Thiamine 1.5 mg

Zinc 15 mg

$\mathcal{W}$eighing Your Portions with a Food Scale

None of us like to wake up in the morning and immediately step on a scale, but if you've never heard of a scale for your *meals*, you might want to reconsider your strong feelings. Food scales became all the rage when bodybuilders and heavy fitness fanatics starting realizing that packaged products often contain vastly different ingredients than what we would assume. It's no wonder that the development of food packaging techniques, homogenizing, and pasteurizing all gained popularity at the same time – whole, fresh nutrients don't last as long as ones that have been artificially treated. Trans fats will last in the milk aisle for days longer than a head of lettuce fresh from the same point. Cooking your meals from home on a vegan meal prep plan will help to ensure that you're calculating accurate amounts for your macronutrients and micronutrients and that you're not overeating without knowing it. Nothing kills a calorie deficit faster than dividing out a Tuesday portion that's much bigger than Monday's. When you're meal prepping and using a food scale, you're going to want to keep track first of all the individual ingredients you've added. You're going to need to use a website with a macro calculator of download one of the hundreds of fitness apps that allow you to upload recipes and ingredients and determine their calories and nutrients. Fan favorites tend to be MyMacros+, MyFitnessPal, Carb Manager, and Lifesum. Each Sunday, once you've finished cooking your entire large-batch meal prep meal, you'll want to make sure you have a large enough empty and dry container to fit the entire meal (these are important details – they can throw off your weight measurements!). Turn on your scale and "zero" it out with the empty container on top. With your meal measured, plug your weight measurement and ingredient details into your app and wait for the total calculated macronutrients. Now, you'll want to have your recipe close at hand, because once you've calculated your entire macro and calorie count, remember that this is for four individuals meals (or however many you've chosen to cook). Divide all your portions out by either even distribution or if you want to be a little more advanced – measure out your portions based on the weight of the entire meal and *the number of calories* you'd like to eat per serving. This method might leave you with extra meals, or fewer meals, but your calorie count will be dead-on, and especially if you're interested in a weight loss deficit, this is the best way to enjoy your meals and not bust your gut.

VEGAN-FRIENDLY FOODS

What to Eat

Veganism isn't just a fun diet for the animals we love and the planet we're trying to save – veganism is a fun diet because it's absolutely delicious! Almost any meal can be made to be entirely vegan, so don't think that missing animal products is going to make you miss out. In the past twenty years, veganism has experienced a HUGE spike in popularity, which means that the pool of creative chefs experimenting with meat substitutes and soy products has quadrupled. You can walk into almost any grocery store and find a hefty number of black bean burgers, vegan cheeses, dairy substitutes, and all-natural (even though they're packaged) vegan sauces. Before we get into those more convenient types of vegan snacks, let's take a look at all the great vegan foods you're going to be eating in each one of your dietary categories. In case you're curious, the vegan food pyramid looks very different from the common "food pyramid," and it's definitely a more satisfying picture to look at. Starting from the bottom, a healthy vegan diet should contain three to five servings of vegetables per day, sticking to green vegetables as much as possible until dinner time. Two to four servings of fruit per day are generally adequate, but make sure you aren't eating four servings of just bananas. Not only are they high in sugar, but you'll also want some variety in your digestion, so you don't get too bogged down in fiber. The second level of the vegan food pyramid is everyone's favorite tasty carbohydrate-packed grain sections. Your rule should always be to stay away from processed grains, but you can indulge in up to eleven servings or whole grains, rice, pasta, granolas, and cereals each day. The third and second to smallest tier is split into two sides, one made up of soy and dairy substitutes, and one made up of beans, legumes, and seeds. Stick to between two and three servings per day of soy alternatives, and between two and three servings of beans. At the top of the pyramid, you won't see any saturated oils, saturated fats, or trans fats. Up at the top are your micronutrients, fats, oils, nuts, and spices. Since these ingredients are much harder to measure in small portions, simply keep it to the minimum amount possible in each recipe. When it comes to finding meat replacements or cheese replacements at the grocery store, keep in mind to check the labels of anything that claims to be 100% vegan. It could be high in sugar, fat, or have hidden animal products. However, some of the best meat substitutes are hidden away in the frozen organics sections, and you can pick up fake chicken nuggets, vegan sausage patties, vegan bacon, and even vegan fish sticks. Although you shouldn't eat too many processed foods, it's nice to know that even a vegan diet has a few cheat options for those nights when meal prep maybe didn't go so well on Sunday. Now that you have a better handle of what to look for when you're grocery shopping and reading recipes, let's take a look at all the things to avoid that you wouldn't know straight away aren't vegan.

· · ·

*W*hat to Avoid

The first and most obvious food group to avoid when you're eating a vegan diet is *animal products*. Eggs, dairy, meat, seafood, and poultry. But it seems like a lot of vegans run into problems cutting out animal products entirely, and that isn't any fault of their own. There are many sneaky animal products that get snuck into our meals without our knowledge. It's one thing to order a steak consciously and deliberately, but if you've chosen to live a vegan lifestyle and get ambushed by something that's against your moral code? That's no way to live. Set yourself up for success by familiarizing yourself with these hidden animal products or animal ingredients. Next time you see them on a label, you'll know to put that item down and warn your friends that it isn't part of a healthy vegan diet. Many vegans tend to miss that any product that contains honey is not a vegan product. If the bee population doesn't survive, then neither does the human population (and agave is a much healthier substitute anyway). But bees aren't the only animals who can offer something to humans that we willingly take.

Plenty of chemical additives in our foods are taken from animals, and if you see chemical formula with a capital "E" in front of it, stay away. Almost all red food colorings, these "E901" indicators on your food labels, come from the scales of insects. You already know that omega-3 fatty acids come from fish and fish oil, but a certain type of vitamin D, called vitamin D3, also comes from fish oil. It also isn't a myth that gelatin is often made from cows and pigs, because their bones help create the texture. While none of this sounds appetizing, you'd be surprised how often we don't even notice that our foods contain an animal ingredient. Any vegan yogurt or cream substitute that contains lactose isn't fully vegan either, because dairy is where lactose comes from. Even coffee and tea creamers that are labeled "vegan" frequently contain animal proteins. The final category of foods to avoid that you should keep an eye on are non-homemade condiments, dressings, and sauces. Many bottled salad dressings and barbecue sauces contain anchovies, bacon fat, sardines, or eggs. Store-bought soups are another animal additive culprit, often using beef broths to make more flavorful vegetable soups or adding ham chunks to split pea soup without noting it on the label. Veganism is all about staying vigilant, but as the months and years go by, you'll learn to immediately identify which types of foods are more likely to have hidden animal products. It's a learning process, but once you've built up a body of knowledge, you'll make fewer mistakes than your peers and cultivate the cleanest possible diet.

WHAT IS VEGAN MEAL PREP

MEAL PREP, short for meal preparation, is a craze that swept the fitness industry in the early two thousand and has proved to be a viable solution for busy dieters looking to track their portions and calories. Mostly used by body-builders at first, meal prep is something that's taken hold in even small town suburban homes with busy families who don't have time during the week to prepare healthy meals. Now that you know how bad processed dairy, cheeses, and grains are for your body, it doesn't seem like a great solution to run through the closest drive through the next time you forget to make dinner. Meal prep allows you to have healthy, home-made meals ready to eat whenever you're hungry so that you don't bust your diet just because you're caught without a nutritious snack. Skipping a meal is just as bad as eating an unhealthy one, and will do just as much damage to the metabolism you're trying to keep high and effective. Plus, cooking your meals at home allows you to see exactly what ingredients, and how much of each ingredient, gets added to your food. Sugars and fats might seem like they're easy to identify, but bad calories are hidden everywhere. Condiments like ketchup and barbecue sauce are actually packed with artificial sugars to give them a nicer taste, and even low-calorie foods that claim to have zero fat are loaded with sugar to compensate for a lackluster ingredient list. Dedicated vegans have also noticed that store-bought salad dressings and so-called "vinaigrettes" tend to be loaded with hydrogenated fats and oils in order to keep them on the shelves longer. A classic vinaigrette is also supposed to be made with olive oil, but watch out for heavier, high-fat oils that have been switched out in order to improve the texture. These dressing are also sadly choked with sugar, and you can imagine the number of innocent people that get tricked into eating way more empty calories than they need. Sometimes, companies will even add egg yolks or whites to their dressings, puddings, and sauces to beef up their constitution. If you aren't the one who's in control of what you're eating, then you might not even know you're consuming an animal product. Taking the time to meal prep before the busy week begins won't just take the stress off your shoulders and help you stick to your diet – it'll prevent you from falling victim to an industry that pays too little attention to what it's producing.

Meal Prep 101

You don't have to love, or even be good at, cooking in order to be good at meal prepping. You'll definitely find that your knife skills will improve as you cut, chop, and prepare meals each week, but don't be intimidated if you don't spend a lot of time in your kitchen. Plenty of vegans survive on takeout from restaurants and grocery store packages, but if you really want to take control of your diet, meal prep is the way to go. Not to mention, the average person who prepares their meals each week saves between one hundred and a whopping FIVE hundred dollars. You might not even be aware of how much extra money it costs you to skimp on the home cooking. Get ready to hit the grocery and watch your pocketbook *gain* weight, while you *lose* it. The main idea behind meal prepping is to cook between one and three of your weekly meals, breakfast, lunch, and dinner before the week starts. Each meal is prepared in a larger batch than one recipe calls for, normally enough to make four portions of the same meal. Now, a word of caution for those of you vegan foodies out there (of which there are many – vegans love to eat!): The same meal for dinner four days in a row is not ideal. We all know it, and the more experience meal prep gurus have learned how to compensate for it. While you won't be tackling this type of meal prepping quite so soon, it's helpful to know that's it entirely possible to prepare your meals and also eat with variety. Normal meal prep days are Sundays, but once you get the hang of it, you can use Wednesday nights as well to create some mid-week variety. In the meantime, focus on prepping either dinner and lunch or breakfast and dinner each week. It's widely known that dinner is the hardest meal for most busy professionals, and even if you only meal prep four dinners in your first week, it will make a difference. Snacks are an easy thing to meal prep if you have a particularly long dinner recipe and need to fill the time in between sautéing vegetables and fully cooking your proteins and starches. But be warned – the more involved your recipe, the more time and pans it's going to take to make. Meal prep is famous for turning your kitchen into a tornado, which is why it's important to clean your workspace and surfaces before you begin. You'll need more than one of each type of pan, so you might want to stock up if you get the chance. Speaking of stocking up, although we'll talk about Tupperware in just a little bit, remember that all this food needs somewhere to go, and if you aren't organized about it, you'll run out of the room. Freezing ingredients before you cook them is a great way to save fridge space and make sure your produce doesn't spoil. Just another way a vegan diet will save you money. Now that you have a better idea of how you'll be meal prepping each week let's talk a little bit about why meal prepping is especially vital for you and your journey as a vegan.

Vegan Prep: Why Prepare Ready-Meals?

Restaurant menus are probably still open on your search history if you've been a vegan for longer than a few months. The food service industry has never been very welcoming to vegan clientele, and even though that's a trend that's changing as veganism becomes more popular, it's still just another facet of how eating animal-free is a challenge in our carnivorous society. Although you might not want to be the person who shows up with their own Tupperware dinner to the company taco night, sometimes, that's just the level of commitment you have to have while eating vegan. Whether you're dedicated to the animal justice side of veganism or to the weight loss and overall health side, you have to decide just how much you care about your results. Now, this isn't to suggest that you should pack up your meals and take them with you everywhere. But there are a few key changes that you can make with specifically tailored meal prep for vegans to maximize your diet. Odds are you don't work from, and if so, you're probably used to the struggle of finding a healthy lunch at work every day. Buy a lunch box and grab an apple, because it's time to start bringing your own again. Bringing your own lunch from home is so much easier if you've taken the time on Sunday to properly portion, cook, and plate your meals. Imagine walking into the office each day and knowing you have a delicious healthy lunch that isn't going to break the bank. Meal prep for vegans doesn't just handle the stress of dinner – it handles the stress of always being hungry but never being sure you'll be able to find the right food. Vegan meal prep is definitely a form of self-care since your veganism is so central to your life-style. It's also crucial to making sure you're getting the right amount of nutrients. Meal prepping is just as important for vegans as it is for bodybuilders – if you don't get the right amount of proteins, fats, and carbohydrates, your body is going to suffer. Using the same equal-sized containers will help you visually see that you measure out your portions evenly. Cooked meat also tends to last longer than cooked vegetables, and so it's easier to leave things like chicken in the fridge and not worry about if it's gone bad. Part of meal prepping is using fresh ingredients and then tracking how long they'll be good for so that you can have three to five days of delicious meals without questioning if they'll make you sick.

Meal Prep Tips and Tricks

No one starts out learning to meal prep and does a perfect job the first time, so remember the steep learning curve and don't put too much pressure on yourself to knock it out of the park. Meal prepping is a skill you'll develop over time, and you'll start to learn how to make more complicated recipes faster and tastier. But while you're just starting out, take a look at these tips and tricks to meal prep like a professional without having to be one.

- Step away from the Ziploc baggies. Vegans are constantly meal-prepping, and if you're using a plastic bag for every single snack you eat every single day, you're going to contribute to the recycling problem just as much as the meat industry.
- Don't forget to use your oven! The stove top is great, but laying out larger baking pans of roasting vegetables will

help you cook more ingredients in a shorter amount of time.

- Include everything you need for each meal in your Tupperware. Sometimes, your meal-prepped meals might call for a lemon wedge for garnish, chopped parsley, or even a creamy sauce. You should definitely prepare these ahead of time as well, and keep them in small containers inside your larger Tupperware.

- Give your spice cabinet a makeover. Meal prep, and the entire vegan cooking, really, often requires you to have more than eight spices at one time. You might be tempted to skimp, but don't! You'll want every bit of these delicious flavors, so make sure you have the right herbs and spices.

- Freezing your meals for later in the week will help keep them fresh, and save your fridge space. Just be sure to thaw them out for a few hours prior to heating up.

- While you're at it, freeze your carbs! Cook large batches of couscous, quinoa, brown rice, and wild rice ahead of time in a pressure cooker and then freeze it in individual portions.

- You can never have enough supplies. Mixing bowls will be in high demand, and if you don't have enough spatulas, it's time to re-up!

- Start with recipes you already know you like. Meal prepping is stressful, and if you start simple with a meal you enjoy cooking and eating, you'll be less likely to quit.

- Don't pour hot soup into a mason jar; pour it into a Hydro Flask! Your favorite water bottle for keeping liquids cold *and* hot is also a convenient place to pour your hot tomato bisque next time you're on your way to work and need a quick container.

- Good food and good friends, make work easy. Meal prepping is time consuming and lonely, not to mention

ELYSE BOSE

kind of difficult. Grabbing a friend to join in on the action will help you manage your workload, and you'll almost always have extras that you can send them home with.

- Prepping for your work out is just as important as prepping your meals. If you're the type that's always ready to hit the gym, make sure you pack up your lunches or dinners if you're going to hitting a session around a meal time. Veganism is all about being good to your body, and if you don't have enough fuel, you won't burn enough calories.

MEAL PREP CONTAINERS MADE EASY

VEGANS EVERYWHERE ARE AIMING to break the stereotype that old ladies are the only ones who get excited about Tupperware. Vegans are constantly taking their meals back and forth from the kitchen to work, to parties with friends. Tupperware certainly isn't a one-size-fits-all sort of situation, and if you already find that space is tight in your refrigerator, you're going to need to do some triaging before you begin to meal prep. However, once you free up your space, this might be the best change you'll ever make for your kitchen organization. Living on a vegan diet means you'll constantly need matching sized and matching depth Tupperware, so invest in a nice set with multiple sets of multiple sizes. You'll want to aim for large sets that have at least four medium-sized containers for your dinners and lunches each week, and you'll need eight total (unless you also prep breakfast, in which case, twelve). Snacks and desserts often need smaller containers, and you can get away with using beeswax wraps (totally humane, and they support the bees!) instead of heavy Tupperware. If you have the interest, many professional meal preppers choose to invest in Glasslock brand self-scaling glass Tupperware containers because of their unmatched ability to keep your fruits and veggies fresh for longer – you'll actually notice a difference. But if you're not set on purchasing an eighteen-piece collection, Amazon has plenty of plastic and glass combination sets that are cheaper, smaller, and will do a very good job. You can also find Tupperware at your local bulk container store, and if you're especially dedicated to weighing your meals on a food scale, restaurant supply stores will have large and cheap containers on top of your scale. If you spend a decent amount of time online, you'll also be able to find meal prep containers that are divided into proper portion sizes – a great solution for all you lazy meal preppers! But keep in mind, this limits the types of meals you can store in that container, and they might not be the wisest investment. Many meal preppers and vegans also like to use mason jars to carry oatmeal, breakfasts, salad, snacks, and lunches. Mason jars fit easily into your backpack, purse, or gym bag, and they seal tightly and securely to lock in freshness without leaking. Just remember to bring a spoon and fork, because there's really no place to put them. Mason jars also come in different sizes, and the largest ones are very effective in fitting classically large vegan salads and lunches. Mason jars can also be used in combination with a flipped upside down empty pudding cup for easy separation between your vegan yogurt and berries and dry granola. Plus, you'll be keeping another piece of plastic out of a landfill. Don't get caught with a delicious meal and no way to take it with you for lunch. The whole point of meal prepping as a vegan is to make sure you're never caught without a healthy, but you're always caught with your morals.

LABELING FOOD

KEEPING Track of Freshness

Pre-packaged foods may be full of things that are absolutely horrible for our bodies, but there's one thing that the food packaging industry got right: expiration dates. Although plenty of packaged foods contain hydrogenated fats and oils designed to last longer than nature intended, their expirations dates are a work of genius. Save yourself the pain and call sick to work when you drink an expired smoothie, and label your meal prepped meals with accurate expiration dates. When you're meal prepping your lunches and dinners each week, the first step to making sure you get the right expiration date for the resulting meal is to double check the expiration dates of your ingredients. If you've just gone shopping on Sunday, you can be sure that all your fruits and veggies, if refrigerated, will last between three and five days. If you've gone shopping a bit before Sunday, you can freeze some of your fresh produce in order to lock in freshness. When you cook your meals, adding ingredients like salt on top to cook out all of the moisture will help your meals last for four to six days. However, you should eat all your meal prepped meals by the end of the week so that you can move on to a fresh new recipe the following week. An easy way to label your Tupperware, either plastic or glass, with expiration dates is to use masking tape. While a sharpie will ruin your container and doesn't wash off, masking tape will often come right off in the wash if you forget to peel it off. While some people prefer to label their meals with the day they were cooked on, others take the time to quickly calculate how many days out the meal is good for, and they'll write down the last day the food is good. Either way, you'll be able to distinguish which foods are past their eat-by date.

Counting Those Calories

If you're in search of a vegan diet for weight loss, the only effective way to ensure you're losing weight is by tracking your calories to create a deficit. A calorie deficit is the most scientific way to calculate how much weight you can lose and how quickly. For the average-sized person, the healthy rate of weight loss is between one and two pounds per week, depending on your height, weight, age, and physical activity. In terms of hard numbers, one pound of fat usually equates to about thirty-five hundred calories. When you're calculating a calorie deficit, it's helpful to know how many calories you need to eat per day to sustain a healthy weight. From there, you can calculate a calorie deficit that equals about thirty-five hundred calories per week, or roughly five hundred calories per day. It's important to note that you should always ask your personal doctor or consult a medical professional before you put yourself on a calorie deficit. You also want to make sure you aren't eating too little calories because this can have the exact opposite effect. When you don't eat enough calories, your body enters into a sort of starvation mode that rewires your storage mechanisms to pack on as much fat as possible for storage, because you obviously need it. Instead of losing weight, eating too little calories often leads to gaining water weight, holding on to unnecessary calories, and a drastically reduced metabolism. This is one of the reasons that it's incredibly important for you to eat breakfast every morning as a vegan. When you sleep, your fasts normally last anywhere from eight to ten hours. If you don't fuel your system for the day ahead, your body won't have the proper energy to carry out your daily activities. Especially if you're dedicated to your fitness, this is a huge issue. Not enough calories mean no energy to work on your physique. Managing a calorie deficit, however, is the perfect way to make sure you're still just as able to work out while you shed unnecessary pounds. Unless you feel that a scale would be an uncomfortable addition to your fitness routine, weighing yourself at the beginning and end of each week is a great way to make sure you're losing just the right amount of weight; not too much, and not too little. Replacing your regular diet with a vegan diet is almost guaranteed to cause weight loss, but for some people, the transition takes a little longer. Don't give up, the results will come – especially when they're supported by a scientific deficit.

RECIPES

VEGAN RECIPES ARE all about utilizing natural spices and herbs to highlight the delicious flavors of natural vegetables and fruits. It's important to keep in mind that vegan cuisine doesn't always have to look and feel like a vegetable. There are plenty of delicious ways to use substitute meat and soy products to give you that hamburger-feel without having to suffer the consequences.

* * *

20 VEGAN BREAKFAST RECIPES

Peanut Butter Banana Smoothie

- 1.0 whole banana, chopped
- 0.25 cups of pumpkin seeds
- 0.25 cups of almond milk
- 1.5 ounces of peanut butter
- 0.50 cups of Greek yogurt

- 0.50 cups of pitted and chopped dates
- 0.50 cups of ice cubes

*P*reparation:

Combine your ingredients in a blender and blitz until you have achieved your desired consistency.

Greek Yogurt and Blueberry Pancakes

- 1 cup of blueberries
- 0.75 cups of low-fat Greek Yogurt
- 6.0 ounces of almond milk
- 0.25 cups of almonds slivered and roasted
- 0.50 teaspoons of almond extract
- 0.17 ounces of lemon zest
- 1.0 teaspoons of whole cane sugar
- 0.50 teaspoons of baking powder
- 0.50 teaspoons of baking soda
- 1 cup of whole wheat flour

*P*reparation:

Combine your entire dry ingredient in a bowl, keeping the slivered almonds separate for garnish. Separately, combine your almond milk, extract, Greek yogurt, and lemon zest. Slowly fold your wet ingredients into your dry ingredients, adding in the blueberries until everything is mixed. Fry over a griddle until golden on either side. Top with slivered and roasted almonds.

Red Pepper Tofu Scramble

- 1.0 whole diced red pepper
- 5.0 cups of cabbage finely chopped
- 0.50 cups of scallions
- 5.0 ounces of firm tofu
- 0.25 ounces of ginger paste
- 0.50 cups of vegetable broth
- 0.75 ounces of sesame oil
- 0.75 ounces of soy sauce
- 0.25 ounces of apple cider vinegar
- Sea salt and pepper
- 0.50 cups of quinoa to serve

*P*reparation:

After chopping your vegetables and warming a medium skillet with sesame oil, add in your red peppers and cabbage. Sautee until crispy, and add in the vegetable broth, tofu, ginger paste, and soy sauce. Add in the scallions and addle cider vinegar and cook until fragrant and crisp. Meanwhile, bring two cups of water to a boil and cook 0.50 cups of quinoa. Serve on a bed of warm quinoa topped with more soy sauce.

Chickpea and Onion Omelette

- 0.25 cups of medium firm tofu
- 0.25 teaspoons of baking powder
- 0.50 cups of almond milk
- 0.50 cups of chickpea flour
- 0.50 teaspoons of curry powder
- 0.50 teaspoons of turmeric

- 1.5 ounces of soy sauce
- 0.50 cups of chopped yellow onion
- 0.50 cups of sautéed cremini mushrooms
- Sea salt and pepper

Preparation:

Warm a medium skillet with olive oil while you combine the chickpea flour, curry powder, turmeric, baking powder, and nutritional yeast together. Add your tofu to the skillet, cooking until warm and seasoning with sea salt and pepper. Add the mushrooms and the soy sauce and cook until soft. Add your dry ingredients to equal parts of water and mix to create a batter. Cook like a regular omelet, filling with onions, tofu, and mushrooms, and seasoning with pepper to serve.

Sweet Potato Breakfast Hash

- 0.50 cups of chopped yellow onions
- 0.50 cups of chopped red pepper
- 1.0 whole peeled and diced sweet potato
- 1.0 ounces of canola oil
- 4.0 ounces of chopped chives
- 0.25 teaspoons of paprika
- 0.25 teaspoons of red pepper flakes
- 0.25 teaspoons of garlic powder
- Sea salt and pepper

*P*reparation:

In a warm skillet with canola oil, sauté your yellow onions and chopped red pepper. In a pot of boiling water, boil your peeled sweet potato until soft enough to grate into hash brown-style shavings. Add the sweet potatoes into the skillet alongside the paprika, red pepper flakes, garlic powder, salt, and pepper. Cook until combined, and then leave flat to crisp in the skillet. Flip halfway through and garnish with chives to serve.

Spinach and Asparagus Vegan Quiche

- 2.0 cups of spinach stemmed and roughly chopped
- 0.50 cups of chopped cremini mushrooms
- 12.0 ounces of drained firm tofu
- 2.0 ounces of garlic paste
- 1.0 ounces of almond milk
- 1.0 teaspoons of nutritional yeast
- 0.25 teaspoons of onion powder
- 0.25 teaspoons of turmeric
- 1.5 ounces of olive oil
- 1.0 ounces of ground flaxseeds
- 0.50 cups of almond meal
- 0.50 cups of whole wheat flour
- 2.5 ounces of warm water
- 0.50 teaspoons of salt
- 0.50 ounces of canola oil
- 3.0 ounces of water on hand

*P*reparation:

Preheat your oven to three hundred and seventy-five degrees. In a large skillet with warm canola oil, sauté the mushrooms until soft and add the spinach, cooking until wilted. Crumble your tofu into smaller chunks and add it to the skillet with the garlic paste, almond milk, onion powder, turmeric, almond meal, flaxseeds, and flour. Stir in the water and canola oil little by little to keep the mixture moist, and then pour into your baking tin. Allow to cook for fifteen to twenty minutes, and then serve when golden and solid.

Vegan Huevos Rancheros

- 1.0 whole all-natural corn tortilla
- 0.25 cups of drained black beans
- 0.25 cups of sweet potato cubes chopped and roasted
- 0.25 cups of drained sweet yellow corn
- 0.50 avocado, sliced and mashed
- 0.50 teaspoons of red pepper flakes
- 0.50 teaspoons of chili powder
- 0.25 teaspoons of garlic powder
- Sea salt and pepper
- 2.0 ounces of vegan sour cream
- 0.50 ounces of chopped cilantro for garnish

*P*reparation:

Preheat your oven to three hundred and seventy-five degrees and warm your corn tortilla. Over a medium skillet with warm canola oil, sauté your black beans and yellow corn until crispy. Add in the sweet potato cubes, red pepper flakes, chili powder, garlic powder, salt, and pepper. When your tortilla has reached its desired crispness, remove from the oven and garnish with your vegetables, avocado, sour cream, and cilantro in layers.

Tomato and Spinach Vegan Breakfast Bake

- 0.50 cups of halved cherry tomatoes
- 1.5 cups of spinach stemmed and chopped
- 1.0 half Yukon gold potato, peeled, boiled, and grated
- 0.50 cups of drained and mashed chickpeas
- 0.25 cups of cornmeal
- 0.25 teaspoons of oregano
- 0.25 teaspoons of garlic powder
- 0.25 teaspoons of saffron
- 1.0 ounces of crumbled feta cheese for garnish
- Sea salt and pepper

*P*reparation:

Preheat your oven to four hundred degrees Fahrenheit and grease a glass baking dish with olive oil. Boil and soften your Yukon potatoes, and then add to a large bowl with your spinach, chickpeas, cornmeal, oregano, garlic powder, saffron, and sea salt and pepper. Mash together to create a hash, and then form into your glass baking dish. Garnish with halved cherry tomatoes with the seeds facing upwards and pressed into the bake. Let cook for twenty-five minutes or until golden and crispy.

Strawberry Guava Acai Bowl

- **For the Smoothie:**
- 0.50 cups of whole still-frozen strawberries
- 0.25 cups of sweetened coconut milk
- 1.0 whole sliced frozen banana
- 1.0 ounces of almond butter
- 0.50 ounces of honey
- 0.50 teaspoons of acai powder
- **Garnish:**
- 1 freshly sliced banana for garnish
- 1 whole guava, halved and scooped
- 0.25 cups of chia seeds
- 0.25 cups of shredded sweetened coconut flakes
- 0.25 cups of pumpkin seeds

*P*reparation:

Blend together your smoothie ingredients in a blender until smooth and pour into a medium-deep bowl. Garnish in sections, leaving the banana, guava, and coconut flakes separate. Garnish with pumpkin seeds and chia seeds.

Cauliflower Chorizo Sausage

- 1.5 ounces of olive oil
- 1.0 whole head of trimmed and chopped cauliflower
- 0.50 a jar of sun dried tomatoes with oil
- 0.75 teaspoons of paprika
- 0.75 teaspoons of garlic powder

- Sea salt and pepper
- 0.50 teaspoons of turmeric
- 0.50 teaspoons of cayenne pepper
- 0.50 teaspoons of thyme
- 0.50 teaspoons of ground cinnamon
- 0.17 teaspoons of oregano
- 0.17 teaspoons of cumin
- 0.17 teaspoons of coriander
- 1.0 cups sautéed spinach to a plate
- 0.50 avocado halved and sliced for garnish

*P*reparation:

In a medium skillet with warm olive oil, sauté your cauliflower with all of your seasonings until golden brown. Add in the sun-dried tomatoes with their oil, and cook until dark brown and crispy. In a small skillet with warm olive oil, wilt your spinach while your cauliflower mixture cools. Form cauliflower sausage patties in your hand and fry in hot canola oil for forty seconds on each side. Serve on top of spinach, with half of a sliced avocado to garnish.

Blueberry Vegan Baked Oatmeal

- 1.0 whole banana, pureed
- 0.50 cups of almond milk
- 0.50 cups of blueberries
- 0.25 cups of blueberries aside (for garnish)
- 0.25 ounces of vanilla extract
- 0.25 ounces of baking powder

- 0.25 cups of maple agave
- 2.0 cups of rolled oats
- 0.50 cups of whole wheat flour
- Salt

*P*reparation:

Preheat your oven to three hundred and fifty degrees Fahrenheit. In a large bowl, combine your blueberries, almond milk, banana, vanilla extract, and maple agave. In a small bowl, combine your rolled oats, wheat flour, salt, and baking powder. Fold your dry ingredients into your wet ingredients, sifting slowly and blending. Once combined, pour into a glass baking dish and bake for ten minutes or until golden and solid.

Chocolate Chia Coconut Pudding

- 0.50 cups of coconut milk
- 0.50 cups of brown sugar
- 0.50 cups of cocoa powder
- 2.0 ounces of vanilla extract
- 0.17 ounces of cinnamon
- 2.0 whole large chopped avocados

Chia Seed Mousse

- 2.0 cups of coconut milk
- 0.25 cups of chia seeds
- 0.25 cups of cocoa powder
- 0.34 ounces of vanilla extract

*P*reparation:

In a small bowl, mix together your coconut milk, chia seeds, cocoa powder, and vanilla extract. Set aside, covered, in the refrigerator. In a medium bowl, mix together your coconut milk, brown sugar, cocoa powder, vanilla extract, cinnamon, and avocados. Let the chia seed mixture chill for four hours before topping with the avocado chocolate pudding. Return to the fridge and garnish with shaved coconut when you're ready to serve.

Vegetarian Toad-in-the-Hole

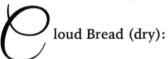loud Bread (dry):

- 2.0 cups of whole almond flour
- 0.25 teaspoons of baking powder
- 0.50 teaspoons of garlic powder
- 0.50 teaspoons of nutritional yeast
- 0.25 teaspoons dried thyme
- Sea salt

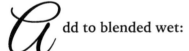dd to blended wet:

- 0.50 cups of almond milk
- 0.50 ounces of almond butter
- 0.25 teaspoons of garlic powder

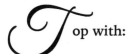op with:

- 2.0 whole carrots peeled and grated
- 1.0 ounces of olive oil
- 4-6 halved cherry tomatoes sautéed
- 0.25 cups of caramelized yellow onions

Preparation:

To make your cloud bread, combine your almond flour, baking powder, nutritional yeast, thyme, and sea salt. Once combined, set aside. In a blender, whip together your almond milk, almond butter, and garlic powder, then slowly blend in the dry ingredients. Once fluffy, use a spoon to layout dollops and bake in the oven at three hundred and fifty degrees for seven minutes. In a small skillet, cook your carrots and yellow onions in olive oil, and then top your cloud bread with both and your cherry tomatoes.

Leek and Potato Protein Pie

- 1.0 ounces of olive oil
- 1.0 ounces of chopped Rosemary leaves
- 0.50 teaspoons of celery salt
- 0.50 teaspoons of onion powder
- 2.0 minced garlic cloves
- 0.50 cups of cubed yellow potatoes
- 0.50 cups of chopped leeks, white and light green sections only
- 0.50 cups of small diced red onion
- 0.50 cups of vegetable stock
- 0.50 ounces of nutritional yeast

- 4.0 ounces of corn flour
- 3-4 whole sheets of gluten-free puff pastry

*P*reparation:

In a large skillet of warm olive oil, combine the leeks, yellow potatoes, and red onion. Sauté until soft, seasoning with salt, pepper, and onion powder. Set aside. Line a greased pie tin with puff pastry and set aside. In a large, deep saucepan, add your vegetable stock, corn flour, nutritional yeast, rosemary, celery salt, onion powder, and vegetables. Cook until the mixture thickens, about eight to ten minutes. Remove and pour into your pie tin and bake in a four hundred degrees Fahrenheit oven for twenty-five to thirty minutes.

Black and White Avocado Toast

- piece of toasted dark rye bread
- Half one avocado, mashed
- Sea salt and pepper
- 2-4 medium-sized basil leaves
- 1.0 sliced heirloom tomato sautéed (or raw)
- 1.5 ounces of balsamic glaze to drizzle
- piece of toasted light rye bread
- Half one avocado, mashed
- Sea salt and pepper
- 2.0 thinly sliced radishes
- 0.50 ounces red pepper flakes
- 0.25 ounces red pepper oil
- lemon wedge for garnish

*P*reparation:

Toast each of your slices of rye bread until desirably crisp. Mash half of one avocado for each toast, seasoning with sea salt and pepper. Dress the first toast with your basil leaves, heirloom tomatoes, and balsamic drizzle. For the second toast, line your avocado with radishes, red pepper flakes, and red pepper oil. Garnish with lemon for taste.

Green Boost Spinach Smoothie

- 2.0 cups of stemmed spinach leaves
- 0.50 cups of chopped celery sticks
- 3.0 large de-veined kale leaves
- 0.50 pear, cubed
- 0.50 green apple, cubed
- 2.0 chopped small carrots
- 1.0 ounces of chia seeds
- 1.0 ounces of pumpkin seeds
- 0.50 chopped frozen banana

*P*reparation:

In a blender, combine all your ingredients and blitz until creamy and smooth, leaving half the chia seeds set aside for a garnish. Add ice cubes for a grittier texture or if you don't have frozen fruit available.

Pecan and Walnut Breakfast Quinoa

- 0.50 cups of chopped and toasted pecans
- 0.50 cups of chopped and toasted walnuts
- 0.50 cups of slivered and toasted almonds
- 1.0 cups of cooked and dried quinoa
- 0.50 cups of almond milk
- 0.50 teaspoons of cinnamon
- 0.50 teaspoons of nutmeg
- 4.0 ounces of maple agave nectar
- 0.25 cups chopped peaches
- 0.25 cups cubed Gala apples

*P*reparation:

In a medium saucepan with three cups of water, cook your quinoa until they pop. Drain and plate in a medium bowl, dressing with your almond milk, chopped peaches, and gala apples. Stir in your nutmeg, cinnamon, and pecans. Then, dress with walnuts, almonds, and maple agave.

Vegan French Toast

- 1.0 cups of almond milk
- 1.0 ounces of coconut oil
- 1.0 tablespoons of whole wheat flour
- 1 loaf of day-old ciabatta bread sliced in 1-inch portions
- 1.0 ounces of maple agave
- 1.0 tablespoon of nutritional yeast
- 1.0 teaspoon of cinnamon
- 0.50 teaspoons nutmeg
- Sea salt to taste

- 0.50 cups of chopped fresh strawberries
- Garnish with maple agave

*P*reparation:

In a rectangular shallow glass dish, mix together your almond milk, coconut oil, maple agave, vanilla extract, and flax egg. Add the nutritional yeast, cinnamon, and salt, and dip each piece of ciabatta bread. Covering both sides, lay the toast down in a hot skillet with olive oil, and cook each side until brown and crispy, about three to four minutes. Garnish with fresh strawberries and maple agave.

Coconut Tapioca with Lychee

- 0.50 cups of toasted coconut flakes
- 2.0 teaspoons of lemon juice
- 14 ounces of coconut milk
- 0.25 cups of black pearl tapioca
- 0.33 cups of sugar
- 4-6 medium-sized lychee, removed from their skins

*P*reparation:

In a medium saucepan of boiling water, cook the tapioca until they pop, then drain. Transfer the tapioca back to the saucepan and add the coconut milk, sugar, coconut flakes, lemon juice, and arrowroot powder. Cook for two minutes on high heat, then reduce and transfer to mason jars.

Top with more coconut flakes and lychee, then refrigerate overnight.

Vegan Frittata

- 0.50 tablespoons olive oil
- 2.5 cups of stemmed and chopped spinach
- 2.0 cups of chopped kale
- 4.0 minced garlic cloves
- 0.50 yellow onion chopped
- 0.50 chopped yellow pepper
- 14 ounces of firm dried tofu
- 2.0 tablespoons of gluten free soy sauce
- 1.5 tablespoons of Dijon or equivalent mustard
- 3-5 chopped basil leaves
- 0.50 cups chopped shitake mushrooms
- 0.66 cups of almond milk
- 1.0 cups of brown rice, drained and cooked

*P*reparation:

In a medium skillet over warm heat, cook your yellow onion, yellow pepper, cloves, and mushrooms until soft. Add in the spinach and kale, and soften more olive oil. Stir in your tofu, seasoning with sea salt and pepper and cooking until soft. Add the soy sauce, mustard, basil leaves, and almond milk with the brown rice. Transfer to an oven-safe glass dish if you didn't cook in a cast iron skillet and broil your frittata in the oven at five hundred degrees until golden brown.

* * *

20 VEGAN LUNCH RECIPES

Vegan Spring Rolls

- 1.0 chopped red pepper
- 1.0 shaved large carrot
- 1.0 shaved medium cucumber
- Roughly three handfuls alfalfa sprouts
- 0.50 cups of shredded cabbage
- 10-12 spring roll papers
- 0.50 tablespoons of cornflour in 1.0 ounce of water
- 40 grams of rice noodles

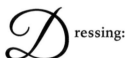ressing:

- 0.50 tablespoons vegetable oil
- 0.50 tablespoons sesame oil
- 0.50 teaspoons of grated ginger
- 1.0 crushed medium clove
- 0.50 tablespoons Chinese five spice
- 1.0 tablespoons of soy sauce

*P*reparation:

To make your dressing, combine in a small bowl the vegetable oil, sesame oil, ginger, cloves, Chinese five spices, and soy sauce. Mix until combined and set aside as a dip. Meanwhile, pack your spring roll papers with rice noodles, cabbage, alfalfa, cucumber, red pepper, and carrot. Use the cornflour in water to seal the edges, and then fry each roll in hot olive oil before serving.

Vegan Crab Cakes

- 1.0 cup of panko breading crumble
- 2.0 cups of chickpeas drained and cooked
- 0.50 cups of chopped red onion
- 0.25 cups of chopped parsley
- 0.50 cups of chopped celery
- 2.0 minced garlic cloves
- 2.0 tablespoons of Worcestershire sauce
- 2.0 teaspoons of fish seasoning
- 1.0 tablespoons of chopped dill
- 1.0 ounces of lemon juice
- 2.0 cans drained and chopped artichoke hearts
- 2.0 teaspoons of mustard (whichever preferred)
- Sea salt and pepper

*P*reparation:

In a large bowl, combine your drained and cooked chickpeas, red onion, parsley, celery, garlic cloves, panko breading, Worcestershire sauce, dill, lemon juice, chopped artichoke hearts, and mustard. Mix everything together, using your hands if necessary. Add in the salt and pepper and shape into patties. Roll in more breading and cook in hot olive oil until crispy.

Vegan Chickpea BLT

- 2.0 toasted pieces of sesame seed bread
- 1.0 whole mashed avocado, salted and peppered
- 2.0 ounces of lemon juice
- 0.50 cups of drained and mashed chickpeas
- 0.50 teaspoons of garlic powder
- 0.50 teaspoons of chili powder
- 0.50 teaspoons of paprika
- 3.0 large green lettuce leaves
- 0.25 cups drained and chopped sundried tomatoes
- 2-3 slices of thin heirloom tomato

*P*reparation:

Mix together your drained and mashed chickpeas in a medium bowl with lemon juice, garlic powder, chili powder, and paprika. Once combined into a creamy texture, start to build your sandwich, beginning with your sesame bread, avocado, lettuce leaves, heirloom tomato, sundried tomato, and chickpea hummus.

Thai Peanut Noodle Bowls

- 6.0 ounces of whole wheat Lo Mein noodles
- 3.0 ounces of warm water
- 0.25 cups of soy sauce
- 0.75 ounces of apple cider vinegar
- 0.25 teaspoons of ginger paste
- 1.5 teaspoons of sesame oil or peanut oil
- 0.25 cups of smooth all-natural peanut butter

- 0.50 ounces of honey
- 0.50 teaspoons of chili paste

*P*reparation:

In a medium pot of boiling water, cook your Lo Mein noodles until desirably soft. Drain the water and warm a medium skillet to medium-high heat with one teaspoon of sesame oil. Add in your noodles and stir. Once crispy, reduce the heat and add in your warm water, soy sauce, ginger paste, peanut butter, and honey. Stir until combined and top with chili flakes.

Vegan Lemon Orzo Salad

- 0.25 cups of olive oil
- 0.50 teaspoons of whole brown sugar
- 3.0 ounces of lemon juice
- 0.50 cups of halved cherry tomatoes
- 0.50 cups of chopped cucumber
- 0.50 cups of preferred pitted olives
- 0.50 cups of drained and chopped artichoke hearts
- 2.0 teaspoons of mustard (whichever preferred)
- 0.25 cups of chopped parsley
- 0.25 cups of chopped cilantro
- 0.50 tablespoons of chopped dill
- 0.50 tablespoons of chopped mint

*P*reparation:

In a small saucepan of boiling water, cook your orzo until swollen and soft, about seven to ten minutes. Drain and transfer into a medium bowl. Add in your cucumber, police, artichoke hearts, and mustard, and stir until combined. Add in the parsley and stir once more. In a small bowl, combine the olive oil, lemon juice, dill, mint, and brown sugar. Stir until combined. Add the halved cherry tomatoes and toss with dressing. Serve cold.

Mexican Kale and Quinoa Bowl

- 1.0 cups of cooked and drained quinoa
- 5-7 large stemmed kale leaves, roasted
- Sea salt and pepper
- 0.50 teaspoons chili powder
- 0.50 teaspoons garlic powder
- 0.50 teaspoons onion powder
- 0.50 cups of chopped and roasted sweet potatoes
- 0.24 cups of drained pinto beans
- 0.50 cups of chopped tomatoes
- 0.25 cups of chopped cilantro
- 0.50 cups of diced cucumbers
- 0.25 cups of diced red onions
- 1.5 ounces of lime juice

*P*reparation:

Preheat your oven to four hundred and fifteen degrees while warming a medium saucepan with boiling water. Cook your quinoa while the oven heats, removing and draining when popped. Meanwhile, grease two baking sheets with olive oil and lay out your kale leaves on one, sprinkling with salt and pepper to taste. Do the same with your chopped sweet potatoes and set in the oven. To the quinoa, add your pinto beans, garlic powder, chili powder, and red onions and stir, then cover and allow to rest in the steam. Once your kales leaves are crispy, remove them and wait for the sweet potatoes to brown. Dress with olive oil to speed the process. Once cooked, lay your kale leaves to create a layer in the bottom of your bowl and top with quinoa mixture. Add in your tomatoes and cucumber and dress with lime juice.

Hummus and Onion Quesadillas

- 2.0 medium whole grain pita rounds sliced in half
- 2.0 ounces of olive oil
- 4.0 ounces of original hummus
- 0.50 cups of pine nuts
- 0.50 chopped and sautéed yellow onions
- 0.50 cups of stemmed and sautéed spinach leaves

*P*reparation:

In an oven preheated to three hundred and seventy-five degrees or a toaster, warm your sliced pita rounds. In a medium skillet over warm olive oil, sauté your yellow onions until translucent, and then add in your spinach. Dress your warm pita round with hummus, onions, spinach, and pine nuts.

Protein-Packed Black Bean Stew

- 2.0 cans of drained black beans
- 0.50 chopped and sautéed large yellow onion
- 1.0 chopped medium carrot
- 2.0 chopped Roma tomatoes
- 0.50 teaspoons of oregano
- 0.50 teaspoons of onion salt
- 0.50 teaspoons paprika
- 0.50 teaspoons of oregano
- 2.5 chopped garlic cloves
- 1.0 halved and chopped celery stalk
- Black pepper
- 1.0 cube of vegetable bouillon
- 0.25 cups of vegetable broth

*P*reparation:

After draining your black beans, warm a skillet over medium to high heat with warm olive oil. Sauté your yellow onion until translucent, then add in your carrot, celery stalks, and tomatoes. Add in your cloves and cook for five minutes. In a warm large sauce pot, combine your black beans, sautéed vegetables, oregano, onion salt, paprika, cloves, and black pepper. Stir in your vegetable broth and bouillon, and simmer on low heat stirring occasionally for at least four hours.

Coconut Vegetable Curry

- 1.0 ounces of olive oil

- 14 ounces of coconut milk
- 2.0 ounces of maple agave
- 4.0 ounces of soy sauce
- 2.0 minced garlic cloves
- 0.50 teaspoons of curry powder
- 0.50 teaspoons of sea salt
- 0.75 cups of chopped sweet potato
- 0.50 cups of chopped yellow onion
- 0.50 cups of roughly chopped carrots
- 0.50 cups of sliced mushrooms
- 0.25 cups of chopped celery

*P*reparation:

Preheat your oven to three hundred and seventy-five degrees and cook your sweet potatoes on a baking tray greased with olive oil. While they cook, in a large saucepan warmed with olive oil, sauté your yellow onions until translucent before adding in the celery, mushrooms, carrots, and onions. Cook until soft, then reduce the heat and pour in your coconut milk, maple agave, and soy sauce. Add the curry powder and sweet potatoes when golden brown and increase the heat to simmer for twenty minutes.

Italian Vegan Minestrone

- 4.0 cups of low-sodium vegetable broth
- 28 ounces of diced tomatoes with juices
- 2.0 cups of diced white onion
- 3.0 chopped large carrots
- 2.0 stalks of celery chopped in lines
- 19 ounces of drained Cannellini beans
- 3.0 minced garlic cloves

- 0.50 teaspoons of dried basil
- 0.50 teaspoons of dried oregano
- 0.50 teaspoons of celery salt
- Black pepper to taste
- Garnish with vegan parmesan

*P*reparation:

Heat a large stock pot over medium to high heat with warm olive oil in the bottom. Once warm, add in your white onions, carrots, celery, cloves, basil, oregano, and celery salt. Stir and cook for three minutes, then pour in your diced tomatoes and juice, Cannellini beans, and vegetable broth. Add in black pepper to taste, using salt only when necessary. Reduce to low heat, stir occasionally, and cook overnight. Garnish with vegan parmesan.

Zucchini and Carrot Lemon Salad

- 1.0 whole zucchinis, spiralized into noodles
- 1.0 whole large carrots, spiralized into noodles
- 1.5 ounces of olive oil
- 2.0 ounces of lemon juice
- 2.0 ounces of vinegar

*P*reparation:

Spiralize each of your vegetables into long spaghetti noodles. In a small bowl, stir together your olive oil, lemon juice, and vinegar. Dress the noodles and serve cold.

Tuscan Bruschetta Bites

- 4-6 toasted 1-inch slices of Italian bread
- 2.0 ounces of olive oil
- 10-12 medium-sized basil leaves, whole
- 0.50 cups of chopped red onion
- 0.50 cups of diced tomatoes
- 0.50 cups of drained and dried Italian white beans
- Drizzle with balsamic vinegar

*P*reparation:

Toast four to six small, one-inch slices of Italian bread. In a small bowl, mix together your chopped red onion, diced tomatoes, and white beans. Add in the olive oil and combine. Dress each toast with basil leaves topped with onions and tomatoes, then drizzle with balsamic vinegar to serve. Garnish with black pepper and salt if needed.

Vegan Teriyaki Jackfruit Sushi

- 0.25 cups of room temperature water
- 2.0 ounces of olive oil
- 20 ounces of jackfruit still in the brine
- 2.5 tablespoons of vegan teriyaki sauce
- Sea salt
- 1 cup of dried sushi rice
- 1.5 cups of warm water

- 1 teaspoon of whole cane sugar
- 1 teaspoon of sea salt
- 0.50 tablespoons of rice vinegar
- 2-4 medium carrots, sliced in thin 1-inch strips
- 1 cucumber, sliced in thin 1-inch strips
- 0.25 cups of black sesame seeds
- Seaweed sushi papers

*P*reparation:

In a pressure cooker, cook and then dry one cup of sushi rice to set aside. In a medium skillet over medium heat, cook your jackfruit with the vinegar, water, sugar, and teriyaki sauce until all the moisture is gone. Add in the sea salt to taste, and then remove. Wet your fingers and roll each jackfruit sushi piece with sliced cucumber, carrot, sushi rice, and black sesame seeds. Roll to complete and seal with wet fingers. Garnish with vegan teriyaki sauce and wasabi.

Greek Vegan Pitas with Vegan Tahini

- 2-3 whole wheat pita wraps
- 0.50 cups of cooked and drained quinoa
- 0.50 cups of chopped and roasted sweet potatoes
- 1.5 cups of mixed greens
- 3.0 ounces of lemon juice (or more to taste)
- 3-4 tablespoons of water for texture
- 1.0 minced garlic clove
- 0.33 cups of ground sesame seeds
- 1.0 ounces of maple agave

- Sea salt and pepper

*P*reparation:

Cook your chopped sweet potatoes on a greased baking sheet until soft at four hundred and fifteen degrees, while warming your pita wraps in a toaster. Boil two cups of water to cook your quinoa. Once popped, drain and stir together with your mixed greens. In a food processor, blend your sesame seeds until chalky and pasty. Combine in a small bowl with your lemon juice, garlic clove, maple agave, sea salt, and pepper. If your Tahini is too thick, add water. Assemble your pita wraps with the roasted sweet potatoes.

Roasted Tofu California Sandwich

- 1 block of pressed firm tofu
- 1 tablespoon oregano
- 1 tablespoon white pepper
- 1 minced garlic cloves
- 1.5 cups of low-sodium vegetable broth
- 1 tablespoon of arrowroot
- 6-8 large green lettuce leaves
- 2 ciabatta rolls cut in half
- 1 whole avocado pitted and sliced
- 1 whole sliced heirloom tomato

*P*reparation:

In a medium skillet with warm olive oil, cook your garlic cloves until fragrant and set aside. Add in the tofu, vegetable broth, white pepper, oregano, celery salt, sea salt, and pepper. Warm, and then add in the arrowroot. As the mixture begins to thicken, allow the broth to boil off. Continue to stir as your remove from the heat and stir in your roasted garlic cloves. On a toasted ciabatta roll, dress your sandwich with sliced avocado, heirloom tomato, salt, pepper, and your onions and tofu. Serve warm.

Vegan Tzatziki and Sweet Potato Bowl

- 4.0 ounces of lemon juice
- 2.0 tablespoons of ground sesame seeds
- 7.0 ounces of water
- 1.0 cups of cashews soaked for 3.0 hours
- 2.0 minced garlic cloves
- 1.0 tablespoons of chia seeds
- diced cucumber
- Sea salt and pepper
- 0.50 tablespoons of dill
- 0.50 tablespoons of parsley
- 0.50 tablespoons of mint
- 1.5 cups of cooked and dried couscous
- 0.5 cups of stemmed and cooked spinach
- 0.50 cups of mashed sweet potato
- Parsley for garnish

$\mathcal{P}$reparation:

To make the tzatziki, combine in a blender your lemon juice, sesame seeds, water, cashews, garlic cloves, chia seeds, cucumber, with sea salt and pepper to taste. Blend until smooth, then add in your dill, parsley, and mint and blend again, tasting for salt and pepper. Once combined, set aside. Cook your couscous in three cups of boiling water, then drain. Sauté the spinach over medium heat in olive oil until wilted while you boil your peeled sweet potato until soft. Mash the sweet potato, then plate the couscous, spinach, and sweet potato. Dress with tzatziki and garnish with Parsley.

Avocado Cranberry Green Sandwich

- 2.0 1-inch slices of whole grain bread
- 0.50 cups of microgreens
- whole avocado peeled and mashed
- 0.50 cups of drained and mashed chickpeas
- 0.25 cups of dried cranberries
- 0.25 cups of pumpkin seed
- 1 teaspoon lemon juice for taste

$\mathcal{P}$reparation:

Toast your slices of whole grain bread with your peel and mash one whole avocado. Drain and mash half a cup of chickpeas. In a medium bowl, stir together your avocado, chickpeas, dried cranberries, pumpkin seeds, and sea salt and pepper for taste. Stir until combined, then dress your sandwich with microgreens, avocado cranberry spread, and squeezed lemon juice for taste.

Spinach and Strawberry Lime Salad

- whole bunch of spinach stemmed and chopped
- 2.0 cups of mixed greens
- 5-7 medium strawberries chopped in quarters
- 0.50 cups of chopped mango
- 0.50 cups cooked and dried quinoa
- avocado peeled and cubed
- 2.0 ounces of olive oil
- 0.50 ounces of water
- 1.0 teaspoons sesame oil
- 1.0 tablespoons lime juice
- Sea salt and pepper

*P*reparation:

In a medium saucepan, cook your quinoa until it pops, then drain. In a small bowl, stir together your olive oil, water, sesame oil, lime juice, salt, and pepper. Peel and cube your avocado, then combine your spinach and mixed greens in one large bowl. Toss in the strawberries and mango with the quinoa, and toss. Add the avocado and dress with vinaigrette.

Middle-Eastern Sun Tarts

- 8-12 sheets of puff pastry

- 0.50 cups of whole cherry tomatoes
- 0.50 cups of purple onion roughly chopped
- 0.50 cups of sliced zucchini
- 0.50 cups of chopped yellow onion
- 1.0 ounces of olive oil
- 0.50 cups of chopped green peppers
- Sea salt and pepper

*P*reparation:

Preheat your oven to four hundred degrees Fahrenheit. Lay out your puff pastry in square stacks of sheets so that you have three sections of pastry and two sections of filling. In a medium skillet over warm olive oil, soften your purple onion, yellow onion, green peppers, and zucchini. Season with sea salt and pepper and remove from heat. Layer your onion mixture on top of the first section of pastry, then top with the middle section of pastry. Line your cherry tomatoes on top of the middle pastry layer and top with olive oil and more pastry. Bake in the oven for fifteen minutes or until golden and crisp.

Southwestern Cowboy Salad

- 0.50 cups of drained black beans
- 0.50 cups of roasted yellow corn
- 0.50 cups of chopped red pepper
- pitted and cubed avocado
- 0.25 teaspoons of cumin
- 0.25 teaspoons of chili powder
- 0.50 teaspoons of garlic powder

- 0.50 tablespoons of lime juice
- seeded and finely chopped jalapenos
- Served cold

*P*reparation:

In a large bowl, combine your black beans, corns, red pepper, and jalapenos and season with cumin, chili powder, and garlic powder. Toss, then add in your avocado and garnish with lime juice. Refrigerate for one hour.

Cilantro and Chickpea Tabbouleh

- 1 cup of drained and dried chickpeas
- 0.50 cups of chopped green bell pepper
- 0.50 cups of halved cherry tomatoes
- 0.50 cups of chopped red onion
- 1.0 cup of cooked and drained quinoa
- 0.50 cups of chopped cucumber
- 0.25 cups of chopped cilantro
- 1.5 ounces of lemon juice
- 0.50 ounce of olive oil
- Sea salt and pepper to taste

*P*reparation:

In a medium saucepan, cook your quinoa until it pops, then drain and set aside. Drain your chickpeas, and combine with the bell pepper, cherry tomatoes, red onion, cucumber, and quinoa. Stir together, and then add lemon juice. Salt and pepper to taste. Serve cold.

20 VEGAN DINNER RECIPES

Classic Vegan Black Bean Burger

- 1 ounce of warm water
- 3 ounces of Sriracha sauce
- 15 ounces of drained black beans
- 0.50 tablespoons of corn starch
- 0.50 cups of grated carrot
- 0.25 cups of chopped green pepper
- 1.0 tablespoons of minced garlic
- 0.50 teaspoons of cumin
- 0.50 teaspoons of chili powder
- 0.25 teaspoons of pepper
- 0.33 cups chopped yellow onion
- 2.0 cups torn whole wheat bread
- 0.75 cups of whole wheat flour

Preparation:

Combine your corn starch, cumin, chili powder, pepper, and wheat flour in a medium bowl and stir. In a large bowl, combine your black beans, carrot, pepper, garlic, onion, and torn wheat bread. Combine, then add in your water and Sriracha and stir. Add your dry ingredients, and when combined, form patties with your hands. Fry on the grill or in a medium saucepan with hot olive oil. Garnish with cilantro or chickpea buns.

Eggplant Vegan Parmesan

$\mathcal{E}$ggplant:

- 2.0 tablespoons of oregano
- 2.0 cups of panko breading crumble
- 0.33 cups of vegan parmesan cheese
- 0.50 cups of water
- 0.50 cups of chickpea flour
- 2.0 medium sliced eggplants

$\mathcal{M}$ozzarella:

- 0.50 cups soaked cashews
- cups of warm water
- 1.0 tablespoons of nutritional yeast
- 5.0 tablespoons of tapioca starch
- 0.25 tablespoons of apple cider vinegar
- 0.25 teaspoons of white pepper
- 0.25 teaspoons of garlic powder
- 0.25 teaspoons of onion powder
- Sea salt

- 24 ounces of marinara sauce garnished with vegan parmesan

$\mathcal{P}$reparation:

Set out a plate of chickpea flour, a flat tray of water, and a plate of breading stirred together with oregano. After slicing your eggplants in medallion-style disks, dip in the water, then flour, then breading. Fry in a large skillet in hot olive oil until golden on each side, about three minutes. For the cheese, mix the ingredients together in a blender and blend until smooth. Transfer to a saucepan and bring to a boil, stirring for two minutes, and then cooling. Pour your mozzarella either into a clean and empty ice cube tray, or a similar small mold that can shape mozzarella balls. Refrigerate for at least one hour. Garnish with parmesan cheese.

Artichoke and Olive Sheppard's Pie

- 14 ounces of drained Italian white beans
- lemon, juiced
- 0.75 cups of soaked cashews
- 28 ounces of drained artichoke hearts
- 0.75 cups of Kalamata olives, pitted
- 2.0 minced garlic cloves
- 2.0 tablespoons of Dijon mustard
- 1.0 tablespoons of nutritional yeast
- 2.0 teaspoons of oregano
- 0.25 teaspoons of chopped saffron
- 0.50 teaspoons of basil
- 1.0 tablespoons of corn starch
- 1.0 cups of frozen chopped asparagus
- vegan pie in puff pastry
- Sea salt and pepper

*P*reparation:

Line a baking dish with your vegan puff pastry after greasing the dish with olive oil. Warm a large skillet with olive oil and cook your white beans, artichoke hearts, olives, garlic cloves, and cashews. Add in the oregano, saffron, basil, and sea salt and pepper. In a medium saucepan that's warm, combine the Dijon mustard, nutritional yeast, lemon juice, corn starch, and vegetable broth. Pour your cooked vegetables and frozen asparagus into the puff pastry base, then add in the broth mixture. Cook at three hundred and seventy-five degrees for forty minutes, covered.

One-Pan Broccoli Pasta

- 0.50 ounces of olive oil
- 5.0 ounces of whole wheat fettuccine
- 0.25 cups of warm water
- 0.50 cups of halved cherry tomatoes
- 0.25 cups of sundried tomatoes with 1.0 ounce of oil
- chopped head of broccoli
- 0.25 cups chopped Brussel sprouts
- 0.50 cups chopped yellow onions
- Garnish with vegan parmesan

*P*reparation:

In a large deep saucepan, heat half the olive oil and water to boil your fettuccine. Cook the pasta, and then drain off half the pasta water. Back on the stove, combine your pasta with cherry tomatoes, sundried tomatoes and oil, broccoli, Brussel sprouts, and yellow onions. Stir together and cook, covered, for twenty minutes. Drain the water and garnish with vegan parmesan.

Best Peanut Lettuce Wraps

- 4-6 large iceberg lettuce leaves
- 2.0 cups of cooked brown rice
- 18 ounces firm pressed tofu
- 0.50 cups of smooth all-natural peanut butter
- 0.25 cups of rice vinegar
- 0.33 cups of soy sauce
- 0.33 cups of sesame oil
- 2.0 tablespoons of chili paste
- teaspoons of ginger paste
- chopped garlic clove

*P*reparation:

In a pressure cooker, cook two cups of brown rice (or a larger amount if you're meal prepping). Drain and set aside. In a medium skillet with warm sesame oil, cook your tofu in small crumbled chunks, seasoning with garlic past and cloves, ginger paste, chili paste, peanut butter, and rice vinegar. Cook down, and then add your soy sauce. Serve with lettuce leaves, rice, and topping.

Spicy Asparagus and Red Pepper Couscous

- 2.5 cups of cooked and dried couscous
- 2.0 minced garlic cloves
- 1 cup of chopped yellow onions
- 10-12 stalks of chopped asparagus
- 1.0 sliced red pepper
- 0.50 teaspoons red pepper flakes
- 0.25 teaspoons of chili flakes
- 0.50 teaspoons of cayenne pepper
- 0.50 ounces of olive oil
- 4-5 large stemmed and chopped kale leaves
- Sea salt

Preparation:

In a medium saucepan, cooked two and a half cups of couscous and then drain. Heat a warm large skillet with olive oil and soften your yellow onion, red pepper, and asparagus. Add in the garlic cloves, chili flakes, and cayenne pepper, and then stir in the couscous as well. Add salt to taste, and remove when desirably crisp.

Vegan Butternut Squash Spaghetti

- 6.0 ounces of whole wheat linguine
- 2.0 tablespoons of avocado oil
- 4.0 minced garlic cloves
- 0.50 cups of chopped yellow onion
- 1.0 teaspoons dried sage
- 1 large seeded and halved butternut squash
- 1.5 cups of low-sodium vegetable broth
- 1.5 cups of stewed spinach
- Sea salt and pepper

$\mathcal{P}$reparation:

In a large saucepan, cook six ounces of whole wheat linguine to your desired softness. While you do so, preheat your oven to four hundred and fifteen degrees and roast half your butternut squash until just beginning to crisp. In a medium skillet, cook your yellow onions until soft, adding in the cloves and stewed spinach alongside the sage and salt and pepper. Take your butternut squash out of the oven and scrape with two forks down the middle to create mock spaghetti noodles. Then, combine in a medium bowl with the avocado oil and everything else. Toss and serve.

Spanish Paella

- 2.0 ounces of olive oil
- 4.0 cups of low-sodium vegetable broth
- 1 cup of frozen artichoke hearts
- halved tomatoes
- 0.50 chopped yellow onion
- 0.50 chopped red pepper
- 0.50 chopped green pepper
- 0.50 cups of frozen green beans
- 0.50 cups of frozen corn
- 0.50 cups of frozen peas
- 1.25 cups of wild rice or Basmati rice
- 0.25 teaspoons of cumin
- 0.25 teaspoons of paprika
- Sea salt and pepper

*P*reparation:

In a deep, large saucepan of warm olive oil, soften your yellow onion, red pepper, green pepper, and artichoke hearts. Add in the rice and vegetable broth, and season with cumin, paprika, sea salt, and pepper. Cook on medium to low heat until the rice has absorbed most of the fluids, then spoon everything into an oven-safe baking dish (if you didn't cook in a cast iron skillet to start). Top the mixture with frozen corn, frozen peas, and green beans, alongside the two halved tomatoes. Cook in the oven for up to one hour or until bubbling and crispy. Garnish with red pepper flakes and chili oil.

Vegan Lentil Soup

- 4.0 cups of low-sodium vegetable broth
- 2.0 cups of warm water
- 1.0 tablespoons of avocado oil
- 1.5 ounces of lemon juice
- 1.0 cups of chopped large carrot
- 1.0 cups of chopped white onion
- 1.50 cups of rinsed brown lentils
- 1.0 cups of boiled and cubed yellow potatoes
- 1.0 cups of chopped celery stalks
- 0.50 teaspoons cumin
- 0.50 teaspoons thyme
- 0.50 teaspoons saffron
- 2.0 teaspoons garlic powder
- 24 ounces of diced tomatoes in their juice
- 2.0 cups of stemmed and chopped kale
- 0.50 cups of stemmed spinach

- Sea salt and pepper

*P*reparation:

In a large stockpot, combine the diced tomatoes and juices, yellow potatoes, chopped kale, stemmed spinach, lemon juice, warm water, and vegetable broth over low heat. In a large saucepan over medium to high heat, cook your white onions until soft before adding in the carrots, lentils, celery, thyme, saffron, and garlic powder. Cook until soft and just beginning to crisp. Add to the stock pot and raise the heat to a simmer, stirring every half an hour for four hours.

Cauliflower Burrito Bowls

- 1 ounce of avocado oil
- 0.50 cups of water
- 1.0 cups of brown rice
- 1.5 ounces of lime juice
- pitted and sliced avocado
- 0.25 cups of yellow corn
- 1.5 tablespoons of taco seasoning
- 0.25 cups of chopped Roma tomatoes
- 14 ounces of drained black beans
- head of chopped cauliflower
- 0.50 cups of chopped yellow onion
- 0.50 cups of chopped cilantro
- Garnish with cilantro leaves and lime wedges

*P*reparation:

In a pressure cooker, cook one cup or more of brown rice. Warm a large skillet over the stove with avocado oil on medium to low heat and cook your onion, cauliflower, corn, and tomatoes. Add in the taco seasoning, lime juice, black beans, and sea salt and pepper to taste. When crispy, serve over brown rice with cilantro and lime wedges.

Stuffed Red Peppers

- 4.0 large stable red peppers with flat bottoms
- 3.0 cups of cooked quinoa or couscous
- 2.0 cups of drained whole chickpeas
- 0.25 cups of sweet corn
- 1.0 cups of stemmed spinach leaves
- 0.50 cups chopped red onion
- 0.25 cups chopped cilantro
- 0.50 cups drained pinto beans
- Sea salt and pepper
- Garnish with cilantro and vegan Mexican cheese

*P*reparation:

Carefully cut off just the tops of your red peppers and find a baking sheet to grease with olive oil that will hold them all. Meanwhile, boil five and a half cups of water for your quinoa or couscous, whichever you prefer. Once cooked, drain and set aside. To assemble the pepper, mix together in a large bowl your quinoa, chickpeas, corn, spinach, onion, cilantro, and beans. Stir together and season with salt and pepper to taste. Fill each pepper, and then seal with a layer of vegan Mexican cheese. Bake standing up in the oven at three hundred and seventy-five for thirty-five minutes. If the cheese begins to brown too quickly, move down one rack and cover with a tin foil bridge.

Spaghetti Squash with Vegan Meatballs

- 1 ounce of olive oil
- 2 tablespoons of tomato sauce
- 1 cups drained chickpeas
- 1 whole flax seed
- 3 minced garlic cloves
- 0.50 cups chopped white onion
- 1 tablespoon oregano
- 1 tablespoon white pepper
- 0.25 cups of chopped parsley
- 0.33 cups of vegan parmesan
- 0.50 cups of vegan panko crumble
- Sea salt and Pepper
- 1 halved spaghetti squash, shredded with two forks
- 1.75 cups of marinara sauce
- Garnish with parsley and vegan parmesan

*P*reparation:

Preheat your oven to three hundred and seventy-five degrees and roast your spaghetti squash until brown and crispy, dressing with olive oil to soften. Meanwhile, cook your onions, cloves, and chickpeas in a medium skillet over warm olive oil. Add in the flax egg, parsley, pepper, oregano, and sea salt and stir. Remove from heat and transfer to a medium bowl to mash, combining the cooked vegetables with vegan parmesan and panko crumble. Roll into meatballs and cook in a clean small skillet of hot olive oil until brown and crispy. Remove your spaghetti squash and scrape with two forks to create long spaghetti noodles. Garnish with warm marinara sauce, meatballs, and vegan parmesan.

Buffalo Cauliflower Bites

- 2.0 cups mixed green salad
- 1 tablespoon olive oil
- 2 tablespoons apple cider vinegar
- 1 tablespoon lemon juice
- Sea salt and pepper
- 1 cup warm water
- 3 tablespoons melted vegan butter
- 1 floret-cut head of cauliflower
- 1 teaspoon of garlic powder
- 1 cup whole wheat flour
- 0.75 cups Frank's RedHot Sauce
- Sea salt and pepper

*P*reparation:

In a large bowl, mix your cauliflower florets with melted vegan butter, olive oil, apple cider vinegar, lemon juice, water, salt and pepper, garlic powder, and hot sauce. Stir until each cauliflower is evenly coated, and then lay out on a roasting rack.

Bake for fifteen to twenty minutes at four hundred degrees Fahrenheit or until crispy. Serve on a bed of mixed green salad.

Balsamic Portobello Sandwich

- 2 large grilled Portobello mushrooms
- 2-3 large slices of heirloom tomato
- 5-7 medium basil leaves
- medium diced and roasted sweet potato

- **Vegan Mozzarella:**
- 1 ounce of lemon juice
- 1.50 cups of water
- 1.5 teaspoons of sea salt
- 0.25 cups of tapioca flour
- 1 tablespoon of nutritional yeast
- 0.25 cups coconut oil
- Sea salt and pepper

*P*reparation:

On top of one Portobello mushroom, stack alternating stacks of heirloom tomatoes, basil leaves, and red onion slices. For the mozzarella, blend together all of your ingredients in a blender until smooth. Then, transfer to a medium saucepan and bring to a boil, stirring consistently. Once boiling, leave for two minutes and then remove from the heat. You should feel the mixture thickening, and at this point, transfer your cheese into either an empty ice cube tray or small Tupperware. Refrigerate until hard, about one hour. Drizzle each sandwich with Balsamic vinegar and add in mozzarella before topping.

Butternut Squash Tacos

- 4.0 ounces of olive oil
- 1 peeled and diced butternut squash
- 1 cup sautéed onion strings
- 2 tablespoons chopped cilantro
- 1 teaspoon of cumin
- 0.50 teaspoons of chili powder
- 0.50 teaspoons of paprika
- 0.50 teaspoons of nutmeg
- 6-8 vegan corn tortillas
- 1 pitted and mashed avocado
- Sea salt and pepper
- 1 cup of white cabbage
- 0.50 cups shredded carrots

*P*reparation:

Preheat your oven to four hundred degrees to broil your corn tortillas. Meanwhile, add your butternut squash to a hot skillet with olive oil and cook, adding in the carrots halfway through. Season with cumin, paprika, nutmeg, salt, and pepper. Remove from heat, and build your tacos with onion strings, mashed avocado, squash, and cabbage. Top with cilantro.

Tomato Basil Soup

- 1 ounce of olive oil
- 0.50 cups of low-sodium vegetable broth
- 1 cup of coconut cream
- 1 cup of chopped basil
- 28 ounces of whole, peeled tomatoes
- 5-6 large chopped heirloom tomatoes
- 1 chopped yellow onion
- 4 chopped garlic cloves
- 2 chopped large carrots
- 2 chopped celery stalks
- 2 teaspoons of dried basil
- 1 teaspoon of garlic powder
- 1 teaspoon of oregano
- Sea salt and pepper

*P*reparation:

In a large skillet, heat your olive oil and sauté the onions, cloves, carrots, celery, and basil. Add in the oregano, garlic powder, and chopped basil, then season with salt and pepper. After you have softened your vegetables, set them aside. In a blender, add your coconut cream, vegetable broth, tomatoes, and vegetables. Blend until smooth and pour into bowls to serve. Garnish with parsley or cilantro.

Classic Mediterranean Pasta Salad

- 1.5 cups of whole wheat rotini pasta
- 1 cups of halved black olives
- 1 cups of pitted and halved Kalamata olives

- 0.50 cups of capers
- 8 ounces of sundried tomatoes not drained
- 0.50 cups chopped red onions
- 0.50 cups chopped cucumber
- 0.50 cups crumbled feta cheese
- Sea salt and pepper
- Garnish olive oil

*P*reparation:

In a medium saucepan brought to a boil, cook your whole wheat rotini pasta until soft. Drain and transfer to a large bowl. Mix in your black olives, Kalamata olives, capers, tomatoes, red onions, and cucumber. Toss, then season with salt and pepper. Garnish with crumbled feta and olive oil – serve either hot or cold.

Broccoli Pesto Shells

- 1.5 ounces of olive oil
- 0.50 cups of low-sodium vegetable broth
- 4.5 ounces of whole wheat mini pasta shells
- 2.0 cups of baby spinach
- 4.0 minced garlic cloves
- 0.50 cups of chopped basil
- 1.5 cups of halved broccoli florets
- 1 cup of toasted walnuts
- 1 cup of toasted almond slivers
- Sea salt and pepper
- Garnish with blanched pine nuts and vegan parmesan

*P*reparation:

In a medium saucepan of boiling water, cook your pasta shells until soft. Drain and set aside. In a large, deep skillet of warm olive oil, cook your spinach until soft, and then add the basil, cloves, and broccoli. Season with salt and pepper, then stir in your walnuts and almond slivers. Once combined, add in your pasta shells and vegan parmesan, and stir until uniform. Garnish with more parmesan and pine nuts.

Edamame Soba Noodles

- 2.0 ounces of sesame oil
- 0.25 cups of soy sauce
- 1 tablespoon of agave
- 1 tablespoon of mild or spicy chili sauce
- 1 peeled and shredded medium carrot
- 2 diced garlic cloves
- 0.25 teaspoons of ground ginger
- 1 ounce of rice vinegar
- 2 tablespoons of toasted sesame seeds
- 1 cup of edamame beans, removed from their pods
- 3 diced green onions
- 1.5 teaspoons red pepper flakes

*P*reparation:

In a large, deep saucepan with warm sesame oil, sauté your carrots, cloves, ginger, green onions, and edamame beans until soft. Add in the sesame oil, soy sauce, agave, chili sauce, red pepper flakes, and rice vinegar – and then add in your soba noodles. Bring the mixture to a simmer, stirring often, allowing the soba noodles to cook and soften in the edamame broth. Once soft, serve broth and noodles together.

20 VEGAN SNACK RECIPES

Traditional Vegan Nut Clusters

- 5.0 ounces of water
- 0.25 teaspoons of almond extract
- 2.0 tablespoons almond butter
- 0.25 teaspoons sea salt
- 1 cup of raw almonds
- 1 cup of raw cashews
- 0.50 cups of candied pecans
- 0.50 cups of chopped dates
- 0.50 teaspoon of cinnamon
- 0.25 cups of chia seeds
- 0.25 cups of hemp seeds

*P*reparation:

In a small bowl, stir together your almond extract, water, and melted almond butter. In a separate bowl, combine the sea salt, almonds, cashews, pecans, dates, cinnamon, chia, and hemp seeds. Slowly fold your wet ingredients into the dry, stirring each time until thick and doughy. Finish by rolling in shredded coconut and refrigerating.

Salt and Vinegar Chip-peas

- 3.0 cups of white vinegar
- 2.0 tablespoons of olive oil
- 2.0 tablespoons of sea salt
- 2.0 tablespoons of black pepper
- 30 ounces of drained chickpeas

*P*reparation:

Preheat your oven to three hundred and seventy-five degrees and grease a baking sheet with olive oil. In a small bowl, combine your olive oil and white vinegar until mostly stirred. Using a medium bowl, combine the chickpeas with your wet ingredients, sea salt, and pepper. Stir to toss, and then pour out on your baking sheet. Cook for eight to twelve minutes, or until crispy golden brown.

Vegan Oat Strawberry Bars

- 1 cup of rolled oats
- 0.33 cups of chopped walnuts
- 0.25 cups of coconut flakes
- 1 teaspoon of cinnamon
- 0.25 teaspoons of sea salt
- 1.5 tablespoons maple agave
- 0.50 cups of soy milk or almond milk
- 1 teaspoon of baking powder
- 1 cup of oat flour
- 0.50 cups of chopped strawberries

- 2 tablespoon of hemp seeds

*P*reparation:

Preheat your oven to three hundred and seventy-five degrees and grease a square glass baking dish. In a medium bowl, stir together your dry ingredients excluding the hemp seeds, while also combining your wet ingredients in a small bowl. Once done, incorporate the two into the medium bowl and stir until uniform. Add the strawberries and stir gently once or twice to mix. In a greased baking pan, pour and shape your bars, then dress with hemp seeds and bake for twenty minutes or until firm.

Homemade Garlic Hummus

- 2.0 tablespoons of warm water
- 3.0 tablespoons of olive oil
- 2 minced garlic cloves
- 15 ounces of drained chickpeas
- 0.25 cups of tahini (ground sesame seeds)
- 0.25 cups of lemon juice
- 0.75 teaspoons of sea salt
- 0.50 teaspoons of cumin
- 0.25 teaspoons of cayenne pepper
- 0.25 teaspoons of paprika
- Black pepper

*P*reparation:

In a food processor, blitz your chickpeas until smooth, adding in the lemon juice, olive oil, warm water, and ground sesame seeds. Pause, then add in your garlic cloves, ground sesame seeds, sea salt, cumin, cayenne pepper, paprika, and black pepper. Blend until creamy, and garnish with paprika, and pine nuts, and an olive oil drizzle.

Banana and Zucchini Walnut Bread

- 0.33 cups of coconut oil
- 1 teaspoon of vanilla extract
- 1 ripe and mashed banana
- 1.75 cups of whole wheat flour
- 0.75 teaspoons of baking soda
- 0.50 teaspoons of baking powder
- 0.50 cups of whole cane sugar
- 0.24 cups of soy milk
- 1 teaspoon of cinnamon
- 1 cup of grated zucchini
- 0.50 cups of chopped walnuts
- 0.50 cups of chopped dates

*P*reparation:

Preheat your oven to three hundred and fifty degrees. Combine the coconut oil (melted) with your vanilla extract, mashed banana, soy milk, and grated zucchini in a large bowl. Mix together your flour, baking soda, baking powder, sugar, and cinnamon until uniform, then fold slowly into the wet ingredients – either using a mixer or a spatula. Add in the walnuts and dates, and stir until combined but chunky. Separate into even bread tins and bake for fifty minutes, or until a toothpick comes out clean.

Loaded Guacamole

- 4.0 large ripe avocados pitted and mashed
- 1 diced red onion
- 2.0 diced Roma tomatoes
- 0.25 cups of chopped cilantro
- 1 seeded and diced jalapeno
- 2.0 minced garlic cloves
- 1 teaspoon celery powder
- Sea salt and pepper
- 0.50 cups drained and roasted black beans
- 0.50 cups drained and roasted yellow corn
- 1.5 ounces lime juice
- Garnish with cilantro

*P*reparation:

In a medium bowl, mash together your pitted avocados until smooth. Stir in the garlic cloves, celery powder, sea salt, and pepper. Add in the red onion, tomatoes, cilantro, and jalapenos and stir in alongside the lime juice. Plate in sections with black beans and yellow corn, and garnished with cilantro.

Overnight Vanilla Chia Pudding

- 2.5 teaspoons of maple agave

- 1 teaspoon of vanilla extract
- 1 cups of hazelnut milk
- 0.50 cups of vegan Greek yogurt
- 4.0 tablespoons of chia seeds

*P*reparation:

In a medium mason jar, mix your maple agave, vanilla extract, hazelnut milk, and Greek yogurt. Once uniform, add the chia seeds and stir. Leave in the refrigerator overnight. Garnish with fresh chopped strawberries, 0.25 cups of hemp seeds, and cocoa powder.

Homemade Vegan Gummies Three Ways

- 1 cup of blackberries
- 1 cup of blueberries
- 1 tablespoon of agar powder
- 0.33 cups of water

- 1 cup of raspberries
- 1 cup of rhubarb
- 1 tablespoon of agave
- 1 tablespoon of agar powder
- 0.33 cups of water

- 1 cup of strawberries
- 1 cup of peeled and chopped kiwi

- 1 tablespoon of agar powder
- 0.33 cups of water

Salted Caramel Popcorn Balls

- 0.24 teaspoons of baking soda
- 0.50 teaspoons of instant coffee
- 0.50 cups of whole brown sugar
- 0.50 teaspoons of vanilla extract
- 0.33 cups of un-popped popcorn
- 0.25 cups of corn syrup
- 2.0 tablespoons of avocado oil
- 2.0 tablespoons of vegan butter
- 0.25 teaspoons of sea salt

*P*reparation:

In a large popcorn popper, pop your popcorn (a deep saucepan with olive oil works well too – if you're not too set on keeping it afterward). Once popped, set aside. Garnish with Himalayan large-crystal salt chunks.

Warm Pita and Red Pepper Bites

- 2-3 warm whole wheat pita rounds
- 1 sliced red pepper
- 4.0 slivered radishes

- **Tahini Garnish:**

- 0.33 cups of ground sesame seeds
- 3.0 ounces of lemon juice
- 1.5 tablespoons of agave
- 5.0 ounces of warm water
- 1 minced garlic clove
- Sea salt

*P*reparation:

Toast your pita rounds until warm, then dress with your red pepper and sliced radishes. For the tahini, blend your sesame seeds in a food processor until smooth adding the warm water and lemon juice to cream. Add in the garlic, agave, and sea salt, and blend until combined. Garnish and serve.

Kale Chips Two Ways

- 12-14 large kale leaves with stems attached

- 3.0 ounces of olive oil
- 2.0 teaspoons of garlic powder
- 2.0 teaspoons of celery salt
- Black pepper

- 3.0 ounces of avocado oil
- 2.0 teaspoons taco seasoning

- 2.0 teaspoons cayenne pepper
- 1 teaspoon garlic salt
- Black pepper

$\mathcal{P}$reparation:

In an oven preheated to three hundred and seventy-five degrees, grease two baking sheets and set aside. Dress your first six to seven kale leaves in olive oil, coating each side, then season with garlic powder, celery salt, and pepper. Dress the other six to seven with avocado oil, taco seasoning, cayenne pepper, garlic, salt, and pepper. Roast for fifteen to twenty minutes or until desirably crispy, turning halfway.

Chocolate Coconut Booster Balls

- 0.50 cups of unsweetened cocoa
- 0.75 cups of roasted almond slivers
- 0.25 cups of melted coconut oil
- 0.35 cups of shredded coconut
- 2.0 tablespoons of flax seed
- 0.25 teaspoons of sea salt
- 1.5 cups of rolled oats
- 1 pound (lb.) pitted and chopped dates

- Cocoa powder and shredded toasted coconut to roll.

*P*reparation:

In a medium bowl, combine your almond sliver, flax seeds, oats, and chopped dates. Mix in the cocoa, sea salt, and melted coconut oil and stir until doughy. With flour on your hands, shape into medium-sized balls and roll in more cocoa powder and shredded toasted coconut. Refrigerate for at least four hours.

Stuffed Dates

- 0.50 cups of unsweetened shredded coconut
- 10-15 pitted dates
- 20-25 almond slivers
- 1 tablespoon of maple syrup
- 1 tablespoon of melted coconut oil
- 0.50 cups of chopped dark chocolate

*P*reparation:

Preheat your oven to three hundred and fifty degrees and grease a baking sheet. After pitting your dates, set aside. In a small bowl, mix together your shredded coconut, almond slivers, maple syrup, coconut oil, and dark chocolate. Gently stuff each date, then fill your baking sheet and cook for five to eight minutes. Cool and serve.

Spicy Black Bean Protein Dip

- 14-16 ounces of drained black beans

- 2.0 crushed garlic cloves
- 1 seeded and chopped jalapeno
- 0.50 cups sweet yellow corn
- 0.50 teaspoons of paprika
- 0.50 teaspoons of cumin
- 0.50 teaspoons of cayenne pepper
- 0.50 teaspoons of sea salt
- 1 ounce of lime juice
- 0.25 cups of preferred salsa

*P*reparation:

In a blender, cream together your black beans, garlic cloves, paprika, cumin, cayenne pepper, sea salt, and lime juice. Remove from the blender and transfer to a medium bowl to stir in the chopped jalapeno and yellow corn. Top with a dollop of your preferred salsa and serve with warm pita rounds and carrots.

*B*lend in a food processor and serve with carrots, pita, and sweet potato chips.

Paprika Celery Snacks

- 4-6 celery stalk halves, cut and cleaned, half open
- 3.0 tablespoons roasted pine nuts
- 2-4 tablespoons of garlic hummus
- 2 teaspoons paprika for garnish

*P*reparation:

Fill each celery stalk, once halved, with garlic hummus. Top with paprika and roasted pine nuts and serve.

Cauliflower Imposter-Corn

- 1 tablespoon of olive oil
- 1 large cauliflower head chopped in even florets
- 0.50 teaspoons of garlic salt
- 0.50 teaspoon of celery powder
- 0.50 teaspoons of taco seasoning
- 1 teaspoon of sesame oil

*P*reparation:

Preheat your oven to four hundred and fifteen degrees Fahrenheit. In a large bowl, dress your cauliflower florets with olive oil, then season with garlic salt, celery powder, taco seasoning, and sesame oil. Bake in the oven flat on a greased baking dish for twenty minutes or until crispy.

Warm Artichoke and Spinach Dip

- 2.0 ounces of lemon juice
- 1.50 cups of hazelnut milk
- 4.0 cups of stemmed spinach leaves
- 0.25 cups of nutritional yeast
- 1 diced medium yellow onion
- 4.0 minced garlic cloves
- 1.5 cups of raw cashews

- 28 ounces of drained and chopped artichoke hearts
- Sea salt and pepper

*P*reparation:

In a medium skillet warmed with olive oil, sauté your yellow onion and garlic cloves until soft. Add in your artichoke hearts and spinach yeast and cook down until soft. Remove from heat and set aside. In a medium bowl, combine your cashews, nutritional yeast, and cooked ingredients. Stir, then season with salt and pepper. Add in your lemon juice and hazelnut milk and combine. Then, pour the dip mixture into either a cast iron skillet or a shallow ceramic baking dish and broil at five hundred degrees for six minutes or until dip is crispy and bubbling.

Vegan Krispy Cranberry Treats

- 2.0 cups of rice crispies cereal
- 0.50 cups of maple syrup
- 0.50 cups of almond butter
- 1 cup of dried cranberries
- 0.50 cups of melted dark chocolate to top
- 0.50 cups of toasted coconut

*P*reparation:

Warm your almond butter and maple syrup in a small saucepan over low heat. Set aside your rice crispies in a large bowl, and mix with the cranberries and toasted coconut. Pour the warm butter and syrup mixture over your rice crispies and mix until sticky and combined. Form into a rectangular or square baking dish for shape and dress with melted dark chocolate drizzles, more cranberries, and toasted coconut. Be sure to press down on each solid garnish just to cement them in place. Keep at room temp and cut in squares.

Mediterranean Falafel

- 4.0 ounces of olive oil
- 15 ounces of drained chickpeas
- 0.33 cups of chopped cilantro
- 0.50 cups of chopped yellow onion
- 3.0 minced garlic cloves
- 0.50 teaspoons of sea salt
- 1 teaspoon of cumin
- 0.25 teaspoons of chili flakes
- 2.0 tablespoons of sesame seed
- 0.25 teaspoons of coriander
- 7.0 tablespoons of whole wheat flour
- 0.50 teaspoons of black pepper

*P*reparation:

If you prefer your falafel to be chunkier, mash your drained chickpeas with a potato masher. If you prefer a smoother snack, blend in a blender with some olive oil. Once done, stir together your chickpeas in a large bowl with the rest of your ingredients. Shape each falafel into a one-inch piece, and fry in a skillet of hot olive oil until golden and crispy. Garnish with parsley and lemon juice.

Vegan Endive and Hummus Rolls

- 7-9 cleaned and peeled endive leaves, half open
- 4-6 tablespoons of red pepper hummus
- 4 tablespoons of crumbled feta cheese
- 5 chopped dates

*P*reparation:

Once you have cleaned and peeled your endives, stuff each one with red pepper hummus, setting a date in the center and wrapping the endive leaf to enclose the date. Seal with a toothpick and drizzle with olive oil and ground black pepper.

10 DESSERT RECIPES

Vegan Apple Cinnamon Donuts

- 2.0 ounces of melted coconut oil
- 0.25 cups of almond milk
- 0.33 cups of whole brown sugar
- 1 cup of whole wheat flour
- 0.25 teaspoons of nutmeg
- 0.25 teaspoons of sea salt
- 0.25 teaspoons of nutmeg
- 0.25 teaspoons of ground cloves
- 0.25 teaspoons of cinnamon

- 1 teaspoon of baking powder
- 1 cup of apple cider
- 1 teaspoon of vanilla extract
- 1 flax egg (1.0 tablespoons flax meal, ground, plus 3.0 tablespoons of water)

$\mathcal{P}$reparation:

In a large bowl, beat your flax egg until fluffy before folding in your melted coconut oil, almond milk, apple cider, and vanilla extract. In a medium bowl, sift together your dry ingredients – whole brown sugar, flour, nutmeg, sea salt, ground cloves, cinnamon, and baking powder. Slowly beat together the wet and dry ingredients, folding dry into wet until doughy. While vegan dough tends to be easier to mix, you might want to use the dough hook attachment on your mixer. Once done, form each donut into a circular shape with a hole.

Key Lime Coconut Bars

- **Crust:**
- 1 cup of rolled oats
- 3.5 tablespoons of melted coconut oil
- 0.25 teaspoons sea salt
- 1.5 tablespoons of coconut sugar
- 1 cup of pecans

- **Custard:**

- 2.0 limes zested
- 0.25 cups of maple syrup
- 1 cup of coconut cream
- 2.0 tablespoons of powdered sugar
- 0.50 cups of lime juice
- 1 cup of raw cashews
- 2.0 tablespoons of corn starch
- 0.25 teaspoons of sea salt

Preparation:

To make the crust, first combine your rolled oats, sea salt, coconut sugar, and pecans. Slowly add in the melted coconut and stir, leaving crumbly but able to be shaped. Form inside the bottom of a greased Pyrex baking dish and bake in the oven preheated to four hundred and fifteen degrees for fifteen minutes. Remove when crispy and let cool completely. For the custard, mix together your coconut cream, lime juice, maple syrup, and lime zest and bring to a boil over the stove. Reduce the heat and add in your dry ingredients (powdered sugar, cashews, corn starch, and sea salt together), slowly folding them into your wet ingredients. Let cool for two minutes, and then pour into your pie crust. Refrigerate for at least four hours.

Vegan Almond Butter Cups

- 1 tablespoon of melted coconut oil
- 0.50 cups of almond butter
- 1 tablespoon of maple syrup
- 1 tablespoon of vanilla extra

- 1 tablespoon of melted coconut oil
- 12 ounces of melted dark chocolate
- 20-22 slivered almonds

*P*reparation:

In a small saucepan, melt together your coconut oil, almond butter, maple syrup, and vanilla extract. At the same time in a separate small saucepan, melt your coconut oil and dark chocolate. Once both mixtures have melted and are hot but not bubbling, pour into any plastic or metal mold lined with a greasing agent or paper. Layer the almond butter and chocolate on top of one another for that classic Reese's look. Top with slivered almonds and refrigerate.

Maple-Glazed Vegan Pumpkin Scones

- **Glaze:**
- 1 tablespoon of cashew milk
- 0.50 teaspoons of vanilla extract
- 2.0 tablespoons maple syrup
- 1 cup of powdered sugar

- **Scones:**
- 6.0 tablespoons of coconut oil
- 0.75 cups of pumpkin paste
- 0.50 teaspoons of vanilla extract
- 0.25 cups of maple syrup
- 2.0 teaspoons of pumpkin pie spice
- 0.25 teaspoons of sea salt

- 0.50 cups of cashew milk
- 2.0 cups of whole wheat flour
- 2.0 teaspoons of baking powder

*P*reparation:

For the scones, combine your dry ingredients (baking powder, flour, sea salt, and pumpkin pie spice) and your wet ingredients (coconut oil, pumpkin paste, vanilla extract, maple syrup, and cashew milk). Blend your wet ingredients in a mixer until smooth, and then fold in your dry ingredients. Shape into crescent moons and bake at for minutes, or until golden brown. For the glaze, combine your cashew milk, vanilla extract, maple syrup, and powdered sugar in a small saucepan and bring to a boil, stirring consistently. Remove from the heat and allow to thicken a bit. Glaze with frosting and serve room temperature.

Cherry Vegan Cheesecake

- **Filling:**
- 2.0 tablespoons of melted coconut oil
- 0.25 cups of melon juice
- 1 cup of coconut milk
- 0.50 cups of maple syrup
- 1.5 cups of soaked cashews (3.5 hours)

- **Topping:**
- 0.25 cups of warm water

- 0.25 cups of maple syrup
- 1 tablespoon of arrowroot powder
- 2.0 tablespoons of lemon juice
- 14-16 ounces of cherries

- **Crust:**
- 0.50 cups of rolled oats
- 1 cups of chopped walnuts
- 1 cups of pitted dates
- 0.25 teaspoons of sea salt

*P*reparation:

For the crust, combine your rolled oats, walnuts, dates, and sea salt in a food processor and blend until chunky. Add in the melted coconut butter and blend again, then shape into a greased Pyrex baking dish and bake at four hundred degrees for fifteen minutes. For the filling, combine your soaked cashews, maple syrup, coconut milk, melon juice, and melted coconut oil in a blender and blitz until creamy. Lastly, make your topping by whisking together your arrowroot powder and warm water. Warm the maple syrup, lemon juice, and cherries in a medium saucepan, adding water to cut if necessary. Once simmering, stir in your arrowroot mixture and remove from the heat, stirring until desirably thick. Pour the filling into the cooled crust, and top with your cherry topping. Refrigerate overnight.

Vegan Blueberry Peach Cobbler

- 1 tablespoon of lemon juice
- 0.25 cups of water
- 0.24 cups of maple syrup
- 1 cup of blueberries
- 4.0 sliced whole peaches
- 2.0 tablespoons of corn starch

- **Cobbler Crumble:**
- 0.50 cups of unsweetened almond milk
- 0.25 cups of melted coconut oil or vegan butter
- 0.50 teaspoons of sea salt
- 1.50 teaspoons of baking powder
- 1 cup of whole wheat flour
- 0.50 cups of coconut sugar

*P*reparation:

Preheat your oven to three hundred and seventy-five degrees. In a medium bowl, combine your blueberries, peaches, maple syrup, water, lemon juice, and corn starch. Mix gently and pour into a greased Pyrex baking dish or ceramic pie dish of your choice. For the crumble, blend together the coconut sugar, flour, baking powder, sea salt, almond milk, and coconut oil or butter until chunky. Pour on top of your cobbler, distributing evenly so that the surface creates a doughy layer. Bake for forty minutes or until bubbling but not burnt. Cool and serve.

Chili Raspberry Chocolate Truffles

- 0.75 cups of smooth hazelnut butter
- 3.0 ounces of maple syrup
- 1.5 cups of dark chocolate vegan nibs
- 0.25 cups of cacao powder
- 0.25 teaspoons of sea salt
- 0.25 teaspoons of chipotle powder
- 1 cup of mashed raspberries
- 1 tablespoon of agave

*P*reparation:

In a medium bowl, combine the cacao powder, chipotle powder, and sea salt. Melt the dark chocolate nibs and hazelnut butter together until soft. Add in the maple syrup, agave, and raspberries, and then slowly fold in your dry ingredients. Stir until combined, then shape into truffles and refrigerate on wax paper.

* * *

Vegan Spice Cake with Baked Apple Filling

- 0.66 cups of canola oil
- 5.0 ounces of room temperature water
- 2.0 cups of applesauce
- 1 teaspoon of sea salt
- 0.50 teaspoons of cardamom
- 1.5 teaspoons of ginger
- 1 tablespoon of whole wheat flour
- 1 cup of whole wheat pastry flour
- 2.0 teaspoons of cinnamon

- 0.50 teaspoons of baking soda
- 1 teaspoon of baking powder
- 0.25 teaspoons of cloves
- 4.0 teaspoons of ground flax seed
- 1.33 cups of cane sugar
- 1 cup of golden raisins

- 1 teaspoon of cinnamon
- 1.5 cups of chopped gala apples
- 1.5 cups of cups golden delicious apples
- 0.50 teaspoons of vanilla extra
- 3.0 tablespoons of whole wheat flour
- 2.0 tablespoon of melted coconut oil

Preparation:

For the cake, combine your canola oil, water, apple-sauce, and ginger paste in a large bowl with a hand mixer. Set aside. Combine the sea salt, cardamom, flour, pastry flour, cinnamon, baking soda, baking powder, cloves, and cane sugar in a medium bowl. Fold your dry ingredients into your wet, mixing as you do so. Add in the flax seeds and raisins after everything has been combined, stirring with only a spoon. Set aside and combine your gala apples, delicious apples, vanilla extra, wheat flour, and coconut oil. Stir until each apple is covered. Lay out on a greased baking sheet and broil for five minutes to caramelize. Pour your cake batter into your dish of choice, and then top with your broiled apples. Bake for thirty to forty-five minutes, or until a toothpick comes out clean. If you don't want your apples to crisp further, cover with tin foil.

Dairy Free Rhubarb Panna Cotta

- 1 tablespoon of coconut oil
- 1 cup of hazelnut milk
- 1 cup of vegan coconut yogurt
- 2.0 tablespoons of maple syrup
- 2.0 tablespoons of agar flakes
- 4-6 vanilla beans scraped of seeds
- 6-7 trimmed and cut rhubarb stalks
- 2.0 ounces of fresh orange juice
- Zest of 1.0 whole orange
- 2.0 tablespoons cane sugar

*P*reparation:

In a medium saucepan, heat the hazelnut milk, orange juice, and coconut yogurt with the maple syrup. Bring to a boil, then add the orange zest and vanilla bean seeds and set aside, covered. Meanwhile, add the agar flakes to half a cup of water and over medium heat, stirring until it begins to thicken. Pour the agar mixture into the milk mixture and stir. In a large saucepan with hot coconut oil, lay out your rhubarb stalks and sprinkle with cane sugar. Candy each stalk, turning so as to avoid burning. Let the stalks cool, and then separate your pannacotta into portions, garnish with rhubarb, and refrigerate overnight.

Vegan Chocolate Cupcakes

- 0.33 cups of avocado oil
- 1 cup of soy milk
- 1 teaspoon of vanilla extract
- 1 teaspoon of apple cider vinegar
- 0.75 cups of granulated sugar
- 0.50 teaspoons of almond extract
- 0.50 teaspoons of baking powder
- 0.75 teaspoons of baking soda
- 0.25 teaspoons of sea salt
- 1 cup whole wheat flour
- 0.33 cups of cocoa powder

*P*reparation:

In a medium bowl, combine your dry ingredients – granulated sugar, baking powder, baking soda, sea salt, wheat flour, and cocoa powder. In a large bowl, combine your avocado oil, soy milk, vanilla extract, apple cider vinegar, and almond extract. With a hand mixer, blend together with your wet and dry ingredients by folding the dry into the wet. Transfer your cupcakes to a lined cupcake dish and bake for fifteen to twenty minutes, or until a toothpick comes out clean.

31-DAY MEAL PLAN

ay One:

Blueberry Acai smoothie bowl

1 whole banana

Thai peanut noodles

2 handfuls of almonds

Squash ravioli

ay Two:

Green spinach and a strawberry protein shake

0.5 cups of golden raisins

Split pea soup

0.50 sliced cucumber with salt and pepper

Sweet potato and leek casserole

ay Three:

Vegan chocolate protein pancakes

1 whole sliced orange

Artichoke Risotto

Carrots with tahini sauce

Mediterranean 3-tomato fettuccine

ay Four:

Vegan yogurt with peaches and walnut granola

5 large strawberries halved

Lemon cucumber mint cold salad

Warm pita triangles with halved olives and avocado oil

Vegan broccoli macaroni and cheese

ay Five:

Vegan French toast

1.0 plum

Lentil and Dijon onion soup

1 whole red pepper dipped in hummus

Mexican-style sweet potato burrito

Day Six:

Open-face papaya granola bowl

Nutty vegan protein balls

Fresh kale salad with lemon and pine nuts

6-ounce chocolate raspberry protein shake

Vegan Alfredo and meatballs

Day Seven:

Vegan Spinach and Tomato Frittata

2 small clementines

Vegan Chinese Salad with Mandarin Oranges

Roasted sweet potato fries

Crispy fried avocado tacos

Day Eight:

Cloud bread with roasted cherry tomatoes and asparagus

1.0 cups of blueberries

Vegan Italian wedding soup

Stuffed dates with feta and almonds

Potato Pierogis with chives and vegan sour cream

. . .

*D*ay Nine:

Overnight chocolate chia pudding with pumpkin seeds

1.0 cups of unsalted mixed nuts

Tomato and vegan mozzarella Panini

0.5 cups raspberries

Vegan pickled okra gumbo

*D*ay Ten:

Caramelized plantains with walnuts and rolled oats

Strawberry kiwi protein shake

Roasted garlic chickpeas with Israelis couscous

Sweet potato chips with hummus

Margherita pizza with vegan mozzarella

*D*ay Eleven:

Potato pancakes with chives and chopped scallions

4-6 halved large strawberries

Garlic rotini pasta with warm avocado sauce

1.0 whole green apple with almond butter

Greek spanakopita with vegan cheese

. . .

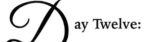 **ay Twelve:**

Maple and cranberry instant oatmeal

Spinach and tomato vegan mozzarella crackers

Brown rice and squash Buddha bowl with sesame seeds

5-Mushroom vegan bow tie pasta

Day Thirteen:

Guava and pear cornmeal pancakes

0.50 cups of cashews

Cream of leek soup

Brussel sprout bites

Vegan curried rice

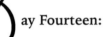 **ay Fourteen:**

Peach and granola vegan breakfast cobbler

2 celery stalks

Warm spinach soup with vegan sour cream

0.50 cups of chocolate covered acai berries

Sweet chili glazed broccoli steaks

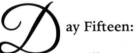 **ay Fifteen:**

Vanilla protein pancakes with maple agave

Orange slices

Cucumber olive and feta skewers

Cajun crispy chickpeas

Carrot and cucumber eggplant sushi

 ay Sixteen:

Dragon fruit and vegan Greek yogurt popsicles

1 whole peach

Vegan cream of mushroom soup

Eggplant parmesan with pine nut breading

Chocolate avocado bites

 ay Seventeen:

Banana vanilla walnut protein shake

0.50 green apple, sliced and dipped in vegan caramel

Glass noodle sesame cold salad

Vegan wheat thins with tzatziki

Middle-eastern lentil and tomato couscous

 ay Eighteen:

Kiwi and Guava overnight hemp seed pudding

1.0 whole pear

Warm chickpea and black bean salad

Mango chutney with warm pita squares

White Bean Vegan Summer Stew

Day Nineteen:

Black cherry and a chocolate vegan protein shake

Almond butter and date cocoa covered protein bites

Pumpkin Seed Salad

0.50 cups of almonds

Jicama and corn lime salad with roasted sweet potato

*D*ay Twenty:

Vegan apple and cinnamon quick oats

Bulletproof coffee with Ghee

Zucchini and basil steamed vegetable pasta

0.50 cups of sea salted almonds

Vegan pistachio loaf with stewed spinach

*D*ay Twenty-One:

Vegan peanut butter and jelly chia balls

1.0 whole plantain

Spicy kale and mango salad

Endives with feta cheese and dates

Vegan Israeli lentil soup

ay Twenty-Two:

Peanut butter and green grape granola bowl

Vegan Greek yogurt with agave and strawberries

Vegan Chinese-style carrot fried rice

Arugula and squash dinner salad

ay Twenty-Three:

Blackberry and lemon vegan protein smoothie

Turmeric latte

Avocado fennel salad with lime vinaigrette

1.0 handful of halved Kalamata olives

Green apple and ginger tofu steaks with peanut sauce

ay Twenty-Four:

Pineapple coconut chia seed acai bowl

Bulletproof coffee with ghee

Classic Mediterranean balsamic salad

0.50 avocado pitted and halved with balsamic vinegar

Quinoa enchiladas with cilantro and tzatziki

Day Twenty-Five:

Half-open granola and coconut papaya bowl

1.0 large gala apple

Vegan jalapeno cornbread bites

Cucumber and dill tahini rolls

Avocado and walnut mushroom ravioli

ay Twenty-Six:
Southwestern grits with vegan cheese and parsley

2 slices of watermelon

Cold potato salad with Dijon mustard

1.0 whole gala apple

Vegan sausage and marinara linguine

ay Twenty-Seven:
Dark chocolate lavender protein pancakes

5 carrots in tahini sauce

Baby spinach and cranberry toasted almond salad

4 Oreo cookies (they're vegan!)

Vegan Dim Sum with soy sauce and ginger

ay Twenty-Eight:
Vegan tofu scrambled eggs with sundried tomatoes

Crispy garlic kale chips with vegan ranch dip

Cream of broccoli soup

2 handful of trail mix

Sweet potato empanadas

 ay Twenty-Nine:

Chickpea hash browns with sesame seeds

0.50 cups of candied pecans

Cold carrot and lemon balsamic salad

Onion and Brussel sprout spanakopita

Chinese style Chow Mein with lentils and olives

 ay Thirty:

Mango and orange citrus smoothie

1.0 sliced dragon fruit with agave drizzle and vanilla protein bites

Brown rice with yellow potato curry

Marinated lime and cilantro cabbage

Green machine broccoli and asparagus pesto pasta

 ay Thirty-One:

Lemon and blueberry vanilla protein popsicles

1 toasted slice of whole grain bread with pine nut hummus and feta

5-nut energy clusters rolled in coconut shavings

Mixed mushroom medley with balsamic marinade

Stuffed Italian pasta shells with mushrooms and caramelized onions

CONCLUSION

Think about the last time you left a fast food restaurant feeling healthy. Now, think about the last time you left almost *any* restaurant feeling anything but weighed down, too full, and uncomfortably gassy. Nutrition in the twentieth century definitely wasn't what it could have been, and we are still dealing with the repercussions of those industry changes today. Pasteurization, hydrogenation, and hormone injection run rampant through the food industry, and all of the most harmful techniques seem to gather around farming; particularly around the farming and treatment of animal products. Whether your journey to a vegan lifestyle began because of your need for a healthier diet, a healthier planet, or a healthier conscience, you've come to the right place.

Veganism has benefits for every single person who commits to an animal-product-free lifestyle, and losing weight is just one of them. With more and more of our daily chemicals and solutions turning out to be harmful to us, there's no better time to step back and start from the ground up. Re-making your entire diet and learning to prepare your meals each week with healthy, whole, vegan ingredients, won't just save you time – it might just save your life. Remember the following list of important health benefits as you begin your vegan diet journey. You never know when a particularly rough day of clean eating might need a pick-me-up, and any one of the many benefits of a vegan diet is enough to fend off a craving.

Eating a vegan diet is proven to be anti-inflammatory, good for swollen muscles and tissues throughout your body, as well as a great facilitator for high levels of good cholesterol. Eating vegan also helps your body maintain a consistent blood sugar that won't experience dangerous spikes, and it may be able to prevent the development of certain animal-product related cancers. Not only that, but veganism is scientifically proven to boost your metabolism, raise your mood levels, promote healthy brain function, and help you lose weight that won't come back after a few years. Eating a vegan diet isn't just about standing up for what you believe in. Veganism and the overall health of the human body are intimately related, and if you promote one, you'll also promote the other. While many individuals are scared away from a vegan diet because of the commitment level it requires, you now know more than most seasoned vegan eaters.

You've absorbed all the information that you need to start creating healthy vegan habits in your own life - but if you're feeling overwhelmed about getting started, don't be! It's absolutely normal to feel intimidated by the wealth of scientific facts that you've just learned. Think back to when you had no idea what "meal prep" meant. One of the first strategies that you learned during our meal prepping section was to take things slowly and break them down into manageable chunks when you feel overwhelmed. That idea doesn't just apply to cooking multiple meals on Sunday night. Veganism is a HUGE lifestyle change, but it's one that's easily done and easily kept forever. Organize your thoughts, organize your supplies, and take veganism one step at a time. It might help to bring a friend along with you – we all know the kitchen, and the workload, is easier with two sets of hands. Congratulations on embarking on your vegan diet journey. Get ready to lose weight and change the world.